The Double-Contrast Barium Meal
A Radiological Atlas

The Double-Contrast Barium Meal
A Radiological Atlas

DANIEL J NOLAN
MB BCh BAO MRCP DMRD FRCR
Consultant Radiologist, The John Radcliffe Hospital, Oxford
Clinical Lecturer, University of Oxford

with contributions by

J O OP DEN ORTH MD *Consultant Radiologist*
St. Elisabeth's of Groote Gasthuis, Haarlem, The Netherlands
W DEKKER MD *Consultant Physician*
St. Elisabeth's of Groote Gasthuis, Haarlem, The Netherlands
B S ANAND MD DPhil *Assistant Professor in Experimental*
Medicine, Postgraduate Institute of Medical Education and
Research, Chandigarh, India. Formerly Research Assistant,
Nuffield Department of Clinical Medicine, University of
Oxford

Foreword by

S C TRUELOVE MA MD FRCP
Reader in Clinical Medicine, University of Oxford

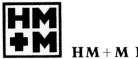

HM+M PUBLISHERS

© D J Nolan 1980

First edition published by
HM+M PUBLISHERS LTD
Milton Road, Aylesbury
Buckinghamshire, England

ISBN 0 85602 072 9

Distributed in the United States of America,
Canada, Central and South America,
Puerto Rico and the Philippines by
YEAR BOOK MEDICAL PUBLISHERS, INC

ISBN 0 8151 6420 3

Library of Congress Catalogue No: 79-56624

Printed in Great Britain at
T. & A. Constable Ltd.
Edinburgh

Contents

Foreword

My major interest in medicine is gastroenterology, in which radiology plays a vital role in diagnosis. It has been my good fortune to have worked in close association with two radiologists with outstanding skill in this branch of medicine. For a quarter of a century, Dr. Kenneth Lumsden was my radiological right hand, but our professional collaboration (though not our friendship) ceased when he retired from the National Health Service.

However, we have been most fortunate at Oxford in appointing as his successor the author of the present book, Dr. Dan Nolan, with whom I have formed a professional association just as close as the one I had previously with Kenneth Lumsden, and with whom I am equally friendly. It is a great pleasure to find that he is constantly seeking to improve the standard of radiological examinations required for the diagnosis of gastrointestinal disease. Among these examinations, the adoption of the double-contrast barium meal as the routine method has proved to be highly advantageous and the present book summarises his experience with the method and his reasons for advocating its universal adoption.

The past decade has seen an immense growth in upper gastrointestinal endoscopy as a result of the development of flexible fibreoptic instruments with facilities for obtaining biopsy specimens under direct vision. Some enthusiasts would abandon the barium meal as the primary method of investigation, but the use of the double-contrast examination enables a selective policy for endoscopy to be adopted, thus sparing some of the patients a measure of discomfort and the risk of complications of endoscopy, which, although a small risk, nevertheless exists.

It gives me great pleasure to express my hope that this book will prove to be a great success and that it will be read not only by radiologists but also by clinicians interested in gastroenterology, as I am convinced that it is an important step forward in diagnostic methods.

S. C. TRUELOVE
July 1979

Preface

The increasing use of fibre-optic endoscopy in recent years has revealed that the conventional barium meal is inadequate for showing medium-sized and small lesions. In Japan, where there is a high incidence of gastric cancer, radiologists have developed and refined a double-contrast barium technique. It is possible with this examination to detect small carcinomas that have not spread beyond the mucosa and the prognosis for such patients has improved as a result. Advantages of the technique are that lesions as small as 3 mm in diameter can be clearly shown. The lesions are shown *en face*, and the mucosal relief pattern closely resembles the endoscopic and macroscopic appearances.

The double-contrast barium meal is now being adopted in many centres as the routine radiological method for examining the upper gastrointestinal tract, and it is well-recognized that it gives much better results than the conventional examination. There are, however, many different methods advocated for performing the double-contrast examination. In this book the development of the technique is reviewed and the materials and equipment involved are discussed. A detailed description is given of one method of performing the double-contrast examination that is suitable for routine use in a busy department. Illustrations of many different lesions which can be demonstrated by this method are included, and the presence of almost all the lesions depicted has been verified by endoscopy or surgery.

It is hoped this atlas will stimulate and assist radiologists interested in the new technique and that it will be a useful reference source for radiologists and for physicians and surgeons whose concern is the diagnosis of upper gastrointestinal disease.

D J NOLAN
July 1979

Acknowledgements

I wish to acknowledge the many people who have assisted me directly or indirectly with the preparation of this book. I owe a debt of gratitude to Professor Middlemiss and his colleagues in Bristol who gave me my training in radiology. Dr Louis Kreel, Dr Geoffrey Scott-Harden and Dr Giles Stevenson kindly gave me the benefit of their experience with the double-contrast barium meal when I sought their assistance following my appointment at Oxford.

Dr Sidney Truelove and Mr Emanoel Lee have given me their fullest support and encouragement and have earned my extra special gratitude. I wish to thank my colleagues in the Department of Radiology at the Radcliffe Infirmary for their co-operation, my clinical colleagues who referred the patients, the members of the Nuffield Department of Clinical Medicine who carried out the endoscopies, and Dr Juan Piris of the Department of Pathology.

The book would not be complete without the contributors who provided chapters in their areas of expertise. My thanks are due to them and to Dr Giles Stevenson, Dr Craig MacLarnon and the editor of *Clinical Radiology* who allowed me to reproduce some of their material. I am grateful to Dr Hans Herlinger, Mr Emanoel Lee and Dr Roscoe Miller who read the manuscript and made constructive criticisms.

I should like to thank the radiographers at the Radcliffe Infirmary and in particular Miss Jean Sangster and Miss Sara Twemlow for providing high quality radiography, and also Miss Sylvia Barker of the Department of Medical Illustration for preparing the line drawings. My wife, Rosarie, typed the manuscript and her assistance was invaluable. I am grateful to her, and to Mr Patrick West of HM + M Publishers who dedicated much time and effort to the production of this book.

1 Introduction

The shortcomings of a conventional single-contrast barium examination of the upper gastrointestinal tract have been recognized for many years. When this method is used lesions are only detected if they cause a change in the outline of the barium-filled stomach. The radiographs thus obtained show the lesion in profile; as a result only medium and large-sized lesions are demonstrated and small lesions and minor changes in the mucosal pattern elude detection. The double-contrast barium meal examination overcomes this disadvantage.

One of the first workers to obtain double-contrast views of the stomach was Hilpert in 1928 who injected air and barium through a nasogastric tube. A combination of barium and Seidlitz powders (which release carbon dioxide on reaching the stomach) were used successfully by Arens & Mesirow in 1937. The use of double-contrast techniques for showing the stomach was also reported by Wasch & Epstein in 1944 and Ruzicka & Rigler in 1951, but the method did not become widely accepted for routine examinations at the time. The increasing use of the double-contrast method at the present time owes much to Japanese radiologists (Ichikawa *et al.* 1966; Shirakabe 1966, 1971) who performed successful double-contrast examinations of the stomach from about 1953 onwards by having the patient ingest barium and insufflating air into his stomach through a gastric tube (Shirakabe 1971). Compression radiography and the filling method were incorporated in the examination.

The high incidence of gastric carcinoma in Japan and the poor prognosis when it was detected by the conventional barium meal prompted the widespread adoption of the double-contrast examination. The results were very encouraging: where previously early gastric cancer was found only by chance, many cases were discovered with minimal and therefore potentially curable lesions. Shortly after its introduction the double-contrast barium meal was modified so that it could be used as a screening procedure in Japan for the detection of early gastric cancer. Since 1956 mass surveys using the double-contrast technique (six films without fluoroscopy) have been carried out (Ariga & Takahashi 1976). The impact of double-contrast radiography was so great that it could be said that there was no hospital in Japan which did not use it (Shirakabe 1971). Since the late sixties the advantages of the double-contrast barium meal examination have been recognized by radiologists throughout the world (Kalokerinos 1967; Heitzeberg & Treichel 1972; Scott-Harden 1972; Kreel *et al.* 1973; Gelfand 1975; Laufer *et al.* 1975; Op den Orth 1975; de Lacey 1977) and it is now replacing the 'old style' barium meal in most centres.

The double-contrast method allows the stomach to be distended with gas while retaining the ability to visualize its inner surface. The gas puts the gastric mucosa under slight tension, and lesions causing lack of distensibility result in a clearly visible series of converging folds (Gelfand 1975). Carcinomas, ulcers and ulcer scars that have a converging fold pattern are easily detected. Small lesions and slight irregularity of the mucosa can be identified. Another big advantage of this method is that lesions are shown *en face*. Thus the size, shape and details of the margin of lesions can be accurately assessed and the radiological appearances closely resemble those of the resected specimens.

While these developments were taking place in radiology, major advances were also being made in the design and manufacture of endoscopic equipment. With the modern fibre-optic instruments it is possible to visualize and photograph lesions and also to obtain aimed biopsy and cytology specimens. By combining their use with X-ray examinations a histological diagnosis of each lesion found on double-contrast studies can be obtained before operation. Success in diagnosing and detecting lesions in the upper gastrointestinal tract is best achieved by close co-operation between the radiologist carrying out double-contrast studies and the endoscopist (Ichikawa *et al.* 1966; Scobie 1970; Kawai 1972; Fevre *et al.* 1976; Dekker & Op den Orth 1977).

In the past many studies have shown endoscopy to be far superior to the conventional barium meal examination. In one such study by Fung & Lee (1976) the authors suggested that the conventional barium meal should not be performed but should be replaced by the double-contrast method — 'Japanese style'. Studies comparing the relative diagnostic accuracy of the double-contrast barium meal with endoscopy show that the double-contrast examination of the stomach and duodenum is highly accurate. In one study 1500 patients with gastrointestinal symptoms were examined by double-contrast gastroduodenal radiology (Laufer 1976) 225 of whom were also examined by endoscopy, and a radiological error rate of only seven per cent was found. Lesions such as erosions, linear ulcers and ulcer scars that could not be demonstrated by the conventional barium meal were identified when the double-contrast method was used. Half the radiological studies were performed by residents in training and supervision was only given during interpretation of the films, which suggests that the mechanics of the examination can easily be learned.

X-ray-negative dyspepsia is quoted as an indication for endoscopic examination because of the inaccuracy of the single-contrast technique but the results of a study by Salter (1977) show that this is not the case when the double-contrast method is in routine use. Of 140 patients who presented with dyspepsia and who had negative findings in the double-contrast study, no abnormality was found at endoscopy in 133. The lesions detected in the remaining seven were oesophagitis in two, antral erosions in two, a duodenal ulcer in two and a chronic benign gastric ulcer in one. It was concluded that the increased accuracy of the double-contrast technique would release endoscopists from the obligation of examining every patient with X-ray-negative dyspepsia and allow them to concentrate on the investigation of radiological abnormalities which need visual confirmation or histological evaluation.

Double-contrast radiology has two big advantages over endoscopy. The first is that each of the X-ray films obtained provides an image of large areas of the gastric mucosa which is available at any time for detailed review, and which can be retained as a permanent record. The second advantage is that double-contrast radiology is quick to perform and much less uncomfortable for the patient than endoscopy, and it should therefore remain the initial diagnostic procedure. Upper gastro-intestinal endoscopy is relatively safe but there are slight hazards associated with it which do not occur with barium examinations. Perforation of the oesophagus may occur in patients with Zenker's or oesophageal diverticula. A prior barium study should identify the patients with diverticula.

Some radiologists argue that a double-contrast examination is too time-consuming and they continue to use the conventional barium meal. As with any new method it appears to take longer when it is first adopted but once the technique is mastered it takes no longer than the conventional barium meal. Radiologists who have adopted the new method testify that it is quick, no more time-consuming than the conventional method, well tolerated by the patient and suitable for use in a busy radiology department (Scott-Harden 1973; Hunt & Anderson 1976; Op den Orth & Ploem 1977; Saxton 1977). As has already been mentioned, the double-contrast technique is used in Japan for mass screening to detect early gastric cancer and this shows that the examination can be carried out quickly while at the same time retaining its accuracy. In 1971 a total of 1,886,062 people were examined in a mass survey and the average detection rate for carcinoma of the stomach was 0·15 per cent (Ariga & Takahashi 1976).

References

Arens R. A. & Mesirow S. D. (1937) *Radiology*, **29**, 1

Ariga K. & Takahashi K. (1976) *Gastric Mass Survey in Cancer in Asia; Monograph in Cancer Research, 18* (Ed. Hirayama T.) Baltimore: University Park Press

Dekker W. & Op den Orth J. O. (1977) *Radiol. Clin. (Basel)*, **46**, 115

Fevre D. I., Green P. H. R., Barrett P. J. & Nagy G. S. (1976) *Gut*, **17**, 41

Fung W-P. & Lee S-K. (1976) *Med. J. Aust.*, **2**, 241

Gelfand D. W. (1975) *Am. J. Gastroent.*, **63**, 216

Heitzeberg H. & Treichel J. (1972) *Fortschr. Roentgenstr.*, **116**, 529

Herlinger H., Glanville J. N. & Kreel L. (1977) *Clin. Radiol.*, **28**, 307

Hilpert F. (1928) *Fortschr. Roentgenstr.*, **38**, 80

Hunt J. H. & Anderson I. F. (1976) *Clin. Radiol.*, **27**, 87

Ichikawa H., Yamada T., Hirikoshi H. & Doi H. (1966) In *Recent Advances in Gastroenterology Vol. 1* (Ed. Ueda H., Harada T., Kameda H. & Tsuneako K.) Proceedings of the 3rd World Congress of Gastroenterology, Tokyo

Kalokerinos J. (1967) *Aust. Radiol.*, **11**, 246

Kawai K. (1972) *Endoscopy*, **4**, 39

Kreel L., Herlinger H. & Glanville J. (1973) *Clin. Radiol.*, **24**, 307

Lacey G. de (1977) *X-ray Focus*, **15**, 43

Laufer I. (1976) *Gastroenterology*, **71**, 874

Laufer I., Mullens J. E. & Hamilton J. (1975) *Radiology*, **115**, 569

Op den Orth J. O. (1975) *Book of Abstracts — Congressus Tertius Societatis Radiologicae Europaeae.* Edinburgh: Churchill Livingstone

Op den Orth J. O. & Ploem S. (1977) *Radiology*, **122**, 530

Ruzicka F. F. & Rigler L. G. (1951) *J. Am. med. Ass.*, **145**, 696

Salter R. H. (1977) *Br. Med. J.*, **2**, 235

Saxton H. M. (1977) *Br. J. Radiol.*, **50**, 610

Scobie B. A. (1970) *Aust. Radiol.*, **14**, 181

Scott-Harden W. G. (1972) *Gut*, **13**, 850

Scott-Harden W. G. (1973) *Br. J. Radiol.*, **46**, 153

Shirakabe H. (1966) *Atlas of X-ray Diagnosis of Early Gastric Cancer.* Tokyo: Igaku-Shoin

Shirakabe H. (1971) *Double-Contrast Studies of the Stomach.* Tokyo: Bunkodo Company

Wasch M. G. & Epstein B. S. (1944) *Am. J. Roentgenol.*, **51**, 564

2 The Examination

The primary aim of a double-contrast examination is to get good radiographs of the mucosal pattern. These are obtained by distending the stomach with gas and coating the mucosa with an even layer of barium. Smooth-muscle relaxants assist by producing hypotonia. The mucosal coating of barium is applied by repeatedly washing the surface with a suitable barium.

No special equipment is required for performing double-contrast radiology of the upper gastrointestinal tract but certain factors help in obtaining good results. To obtain radiographs with good mucosal detail the exposure time should be short, otherwise there will be blurring due to respiratory movement or to transmitted pulsations from the aorta. Although the contrast of the mucosal pattern is enhanced by taking films at a low kilovoltage it is more important to obtain a sharp image by using a medium kilovoltage (90–110 Kv). With the recently introduced rare earth and barium fluoro-chloride screens, which are about four times faster than the fast tungstate screens, it is possible to obtain a sharp image at low kilovoltage (80–90 Kv). Another important factor in obtaining a sharp image is the size of the focal spot of the X-ray tube, a small focal spot of between 0·3 mm and 0·6 mm giving the best images with the under-couch tube table.

The barium for double-contrast meals should be of medium density and low viscosity. Suitable barium concentrations range from 82·5 w/v per cent (Op den Orth & Ploem 1977) to 100 w/v per cent (Kreel *et al.* 1973). These bariums are best because on the one hand they give good mucosal coating and on the other the density of the barium is suitable for the compression part of the technique.

Gas may be introduced into the stomach in a number of ways. Nasogastric intubation was used initially (Shirakabe 1971), but it is unsuitable for routine use and has been replaced by effervescent agents. James *et al.* (1976) carried out a survey to compare the following techniques for introducing gas: effervescent powder, aerated tonic water, effervescent tablets, transnasal intubation and swallowed air. Effervescent tablets proved to be the best and their use produced a significant improvement in gastric mucosal coating and less bubble formation than the other methods. Another technique for introducing gas into the stomach, the 'bubbly barium' method (Pochaczevski 1973; Op den Orth & Ploem 1977), results in an excellent demonstration of the mucosal detail. Refrigerated barium is put in a soda-making dispenser, carbon dioxide cartridges are attached to the syphon and the gas is released slowly into the barium. One part of barium suspension can absorb two parts of carbon dioxide by volume.

It is necessary to use smooth-muscle relaxants so that the stomach and duodenum can be examined in a hypotonic or relaxed state to ensure that small lesions in the mucosa will show up. An additional advantage is that there is a delay before the barium passes into the jejunal loops where it tends to obscure the stomach. Hyoscine butylbromide (Buscopan) and glucagon are widely used for this purpose and are generally safe and effective agents (Barrowman 1975). Hyoscine butylbromide is an anticholinergic alkaloid which reduces gastrointestinal motility and secretion. Unwanted side-effects associated with its use are transient loss of accomodation, difficulty in micturition, mydriasis, tachycardia, dry mouth, headache and malaise. Additive parasympatholytic action occurs with tricyclic antidepressives and with anticholinergic components of certain 'cold cures' and travel sickness preparations (Barrowman 1975). Massive gastric dilatation is a rare complication. Contraindications to its use are cardiac failure, angina pectoris, prostatism and glaucoma. The dose normally used for the double-contrast meal — 20 mg injected intravenously — would be unlikely to aggravate heart failure or angina. Its action is short-lived, accommodation should have returned to normal within an hour of the injection but patients should not drive for several hours.

Glucagon, a straight-chain polypeptide derived from the alpha cells of the pancreatic islets of Langerhans, inhibits gastrointestinal motility. It is now used in many centres as an agent for producing gastric and duodenal hypotonia (Chernish et al. 1972; Miller et al. 1974; Kreel 1975). Satisfactory stomach, duodenal and small bowel hypotonicity can be obtained with 0·25–0·5 mg of glucagon given intravenously (Miller et al. 1978). Nausea and vomiting can occur but are rare with the small dose used for the double-contrast meal. Glucagon can provoke severe hypertension in patients with a phaeochromocytoma, and sensitization reactions can occur, although they are rare. Even small doses may cause marked relaxation of the lower oesophageal sphincter and make it difficult to interpret the significance of gastro-oesophageal reflux if it occurs (Jaffer et al. 1974).

Each radiologist will want to develop his own particular technique for the double-contrast barium meal examination. The examination should include views of all areas of the stomach coated with barium and the mucosal pattern outlined with gas. Adequate views of the oesophagus and duodenum are also required. It is essential that the method adopted be quick to perform and reproducible. The technique described here is one such method, based on methods that have previously been described (Shirakabe 1971; Kreel et al. 1973).

The patient should be fasting. A short history is taken and the patient is given an intravenous injection of 0·25 mg of glucagon. The effervescent tablets, about enough to produce 300–400 cc of gas are taken by the patient and washed down with 10 ml of water containing an anti-foaming agent. The patient then drinks 50 ml of barium suspension and lies in a prone position on the table which is horizontal. A film is taken in this position at a high kilovoltage to show the anterior wall of the stomach (Fig. 2.1). After drinking a further 150–200 ml of barium the patient first lies on his right side, then turns over on to the left side and finally back to the supine position. A film of the whole stomach is then taken at a medium kilovoltage (Fig. 2.2). The mucosal pattern of the body and antrum is shown on this view. The mucosa of the antrum and body is again washed with barium by rotating the patient as before and a radiograph is obtained in the right anterior oblique position. On this film a good view of the mucosal pattern of the antrum of the stomach is obtained (Fig. 2.3). A left anterior oblique view is taken to show the mucosa of the upper part of the body of the stomach and the fundus (Fig. 2.4).

The top of the table is tilted up to an angle of 45° and a mucosal view of the fundus is taken with the patient either in the supine left anterior oblique or the prone left posterior oblique position (Fig. 2.5). If barium has passed into the duodenum by this stage views of the duodenal cap are obtained. Double-contrast spot views are taken with the patient in the right anterior oblique position either supine or with the head of the table elevated. A prone view of the duodenal cap is taken to show the anterior wall. In many cases it is impossible to obtain a double-contrast view in this position and a single-contrast view is taken instead. Further spot views of the duodenal cap may be taken in the standing position. A single-contrast view of the stomach is taken with the patient standing straight or rotated slightly into the right anterior oblique position to show the incisura angularis (Fig. 2.7). Coned views of any suspicious area are taken but no further views of the stomach are necessary. Compression is applied to the lesser curve and antrum of the stomach in the standing position but films are taken only if an abnormal feature is recognized fluoroscopically. Protuberant lesions are often shown this way. A good compression pattern cannot be obtained unless the lesions are fluoroscopically recognized (Higurashi & Ito 1971).

Views of the oesophagus may be taken in the usual manner at the beginning of the examination with the patient lying in the prone oblique position. However, if the patient has symptoms suggestive of an oesophageal lesion then, of course, the initial mouthful of barium should be swallowed with the patient standing and the oesophagus observed fluoroscopically in case an obstructive lesion is present. Air-contrast studies of the oesophagus are best carried out when the examination of the stomach is completed. Good double-contrast views of the whole oesophagus can be obtained by getting the patient to drink the barium suspension while standing and holding his nose so that large amounts of air are swallowed with the barium. The swallowed air distends the oesophagus and the barium forms a coating on the walls (Figs. 2.9, 2.10, 2.11).

Another useful technique for obtaining double-contrast views of the oesophagus described by Goldstein & Dodd (1976) depends upon the patient taking successive swallows of barium suspension and water and is a modification of the method previously described by Brombart (1961). The examination is carried out with the patient standing, holding a cup in each hand, one containing barium and the other water. The patient swallows a mouthful of barium and follows it immediately with a mouthful of water. Double-contrast views of the whole oesophagus can then be obtained.

Some modifications to the double-contrast technique are necessary in patients who have had previous gastric surgery. In patients with a Billroth I partial gastrectomy the examination is similar to the double-contrast study except that a smaller quantity of barium is used. Further quantities of effervescent agent and barium may be required during the examination as gas and barium escape rapidly through the anastomosis into the small intestine. It is necessary to outline the afferent loop in patients with a Polya or Billroth II gastrectomy. This is achieved by getting the patient to drink the barium suspension while lying on his right side with the head of the table slightly elevated (Op den Orth 1977). When the barium has passed into the afferent loop the table is returned to the horizontal position. The patient then turns into the right anterior oblique position so that gas passes into the afferent loop. Radiographs of the afferent loop are obtained in the supine right anterior oblique and prone positions.

Most anterior wall lesions are detected during the standard double-contrast examination; the initial prone film and the compression part of the examination are important in this respect. A recent study showed that only four per cent of gastric lesions were present on the anterior wall (Goldsmith *et al.* 1976) and it was concluded that the low diagnostic yield did not justify special views of the anterior wall as part of the routine study. However, if a lesion of the anterior wall is suspected a separate double-contrast examination may be necessary. A technique for examining the anterior wall of the stomach was described by Goldsmith *et al.* (1976). An intravenous injection of 0·25 mg of glucagon is given and the patient takes 30 ml of barium suspension and enough effervescent tablets to produce about 200 ml of gas. Coating of the anterior wall is obtained by placing the patient prone and rotating him back and forth into high degrees of obliquity: he is then placed in a 15°-Trendelenburg position with the right side elevated and a compression pad under the left side to prevent excessive pooling of barium. The patient is slowly returned to the prone position and a double-contrast view of the antrum is taken. The head of the table is raised until the body of the stomach is distended with gas and a double-contrast view of the anterior wall of the body is obtained. The prone semi-erect view shows the upper anterior wall. After obtaining the anterior wall views it is possible to proceed to carry out a full double-contrast examination in the usual manner.

The duodenum as far as the ligament of Treitz should be shown on at least one view during the double-contrast examination. When using hypotonic agents routinely for the examination of the stomach it is often possible to get good double-contrast views of the whole duodenum. This is particularly so if there is some narrowing of the duodenum causing delay in the passage of contrast medium. If the radiologist's primary interest is the duodenum, hypotonic duodenography should be carried out and this is best performed as a separate study. Adequate views of the duodenum can be obtained in many cases by the tubeless method. The barium suspension and effervescent agent are taken first and the smooth muscle relaxant is injected intravenously when barium is present in the duodenum. However, the intubation method gives consistently better results than the tubeless, particularly in the investigation of suspected pancreatic lesions. The best projections for showing the duodenal loop can be judged on fluoroscopy and are normally the supine right anterior oblique or the prone position with the patient lying on a compression pad. The proximal duodenum is often shown best with the head of the table elevated about 45–60°.

Patients who are not fit enough to stand while undergoing double-contrast studies can be examined lying in a horizontal position with relatively good results.

References

Barrowman J. (1975) In *The Double-Contrast Barium Meal. Proceedings of a Seminar.* Rickmansworth: Concept Pharmaceuticals

Brombart M. (1961) *Clinical Radiology of the Oesophagus.* Bristol: John Wright & Sons

Chernish S. M., Miller R. E., Rosenak B. D. & Scholz N. E. (1972) *Gastroenterology,* **63**, 392

Goldsmith M. R., Paul R. E. Jr., Poplack W. E., Moore J. P., Matsue H. & Bloom S. (1976) *Am. J. Roentgenol.,* **126**, 1159

Goldstein H. M. & Dodd G. D. (1976) *Gastrointest. Radiol.,* **1**, 3

Higurashi K. & Ito T. (1971) In *Double-Contrast Studies of the Stomach.* (Ed. Shirakabe H.) Tokyo: Bunkodo Company

Jaffer S. S., Makhlouf G. M., Schorr B. A. & Zfass A. M. (1974) *Gastroenterology,* **67**, 42

James W. B., McCreath G., Sutherland G. R. & McDonald M. (1976) *Clin. Radiol.,* **27**, 99

Kreel L., Herlinger H. & Glanville J. (1973) *Clin. Radiol.,* **24**, 307

Kreel L. (1975) *Br. J. Radiol.,* **48**, 691

Miller R. E., Chernish S. M., Brunelle R. L. & Rosenak B. D. (1978) *Radiology,* **127**, 55

Miller R. E., Chernish S. M., Skucas J., Rosenak B. D. & Rodda B. E. (1974) *Am. J. Roentgenol.,* **121**, 264

Nakajima T. & Yoshida S. (1971) In *Double-Contrast Studies of the Stomach.* (Ed. Shirakabe H.) Tokyo: Bunkodo Company

Op den Orth J. O. (1977) *Gastrointest. Radiol.,* **2**, 1

Op den Orth O. & Ploem S. (1977) *Radiology,* **122**, 530

Pochaczevski R. (1973) *Radiology,* **107**, 461

Shirakabe H. (1971) *Double-Contrast Studies of the Stomach.* Tokyo: Bunkodo Company

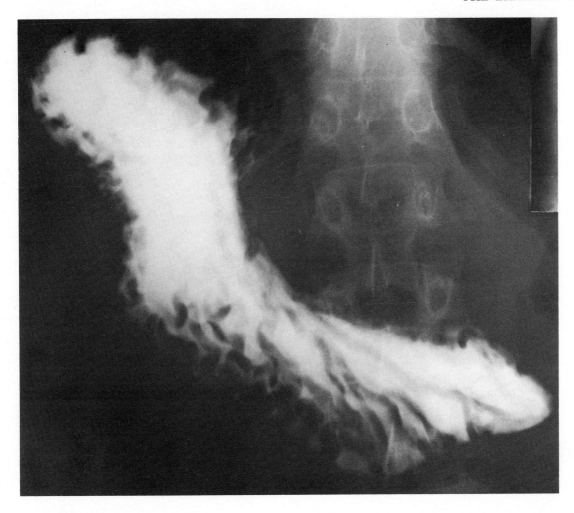

2.1 *Single-contrast prone* view showing the anterior wall of the stomach

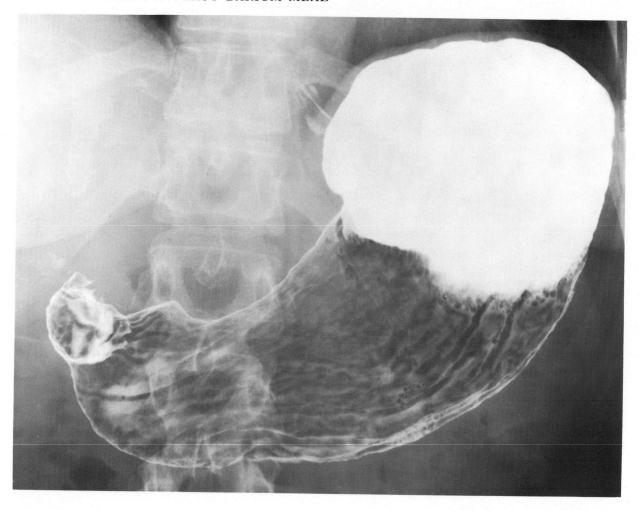

2.2 *Supine double-contrast* view showing the lower body and proximal part of the antrum of the stomach

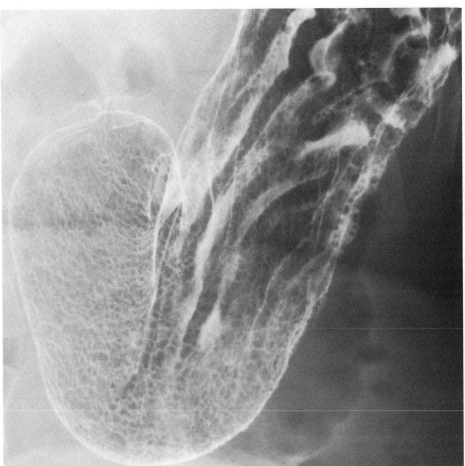

2.3 *Supine right anterior oblique* view showing the antrum and body of the stomach; the areae gastricae are well outlined

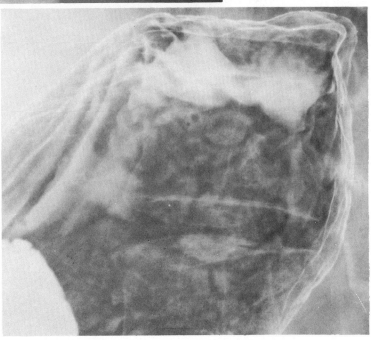

2.4 *Supine left anterior oblique* view showing the upper body and fundus of the stomach

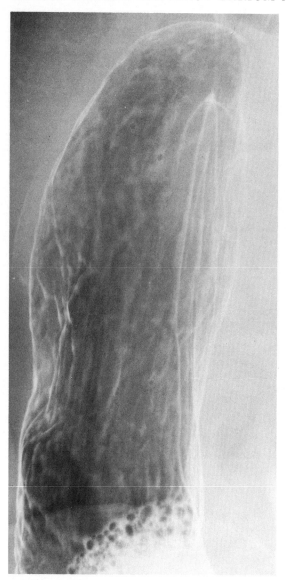

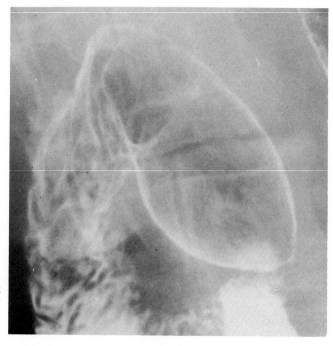

2.5 *Prone oblique* view with the head of the table tilted to 45° showing the fundus and upper body of the stomach

2.6 *Supine oblique double-contrast* view of the duodenal cap

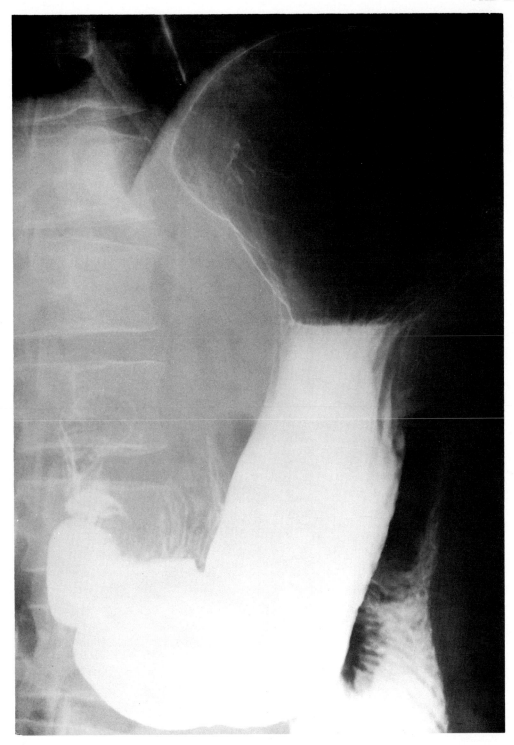

2.7 *Erect single-contrast* view

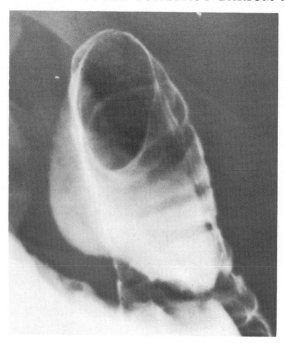

2.8 *Prone oblique double-contrast* view of
the duodenal cap

2.9–11 *Double-contrast* views of the
oesophagus

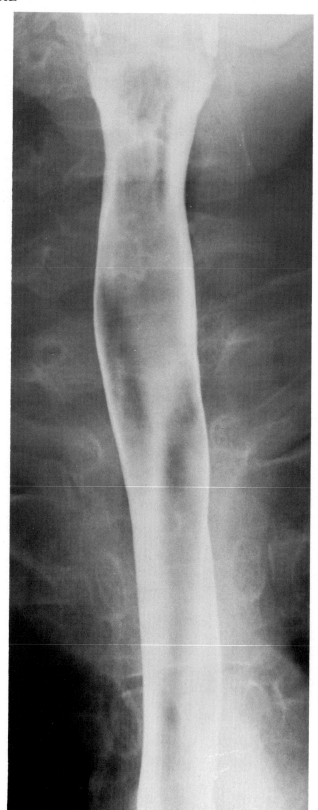

2.9

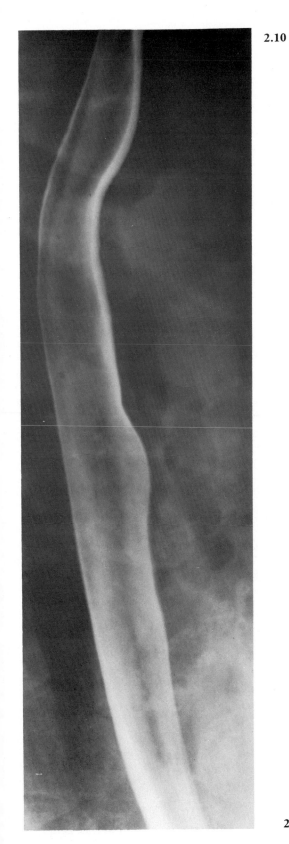

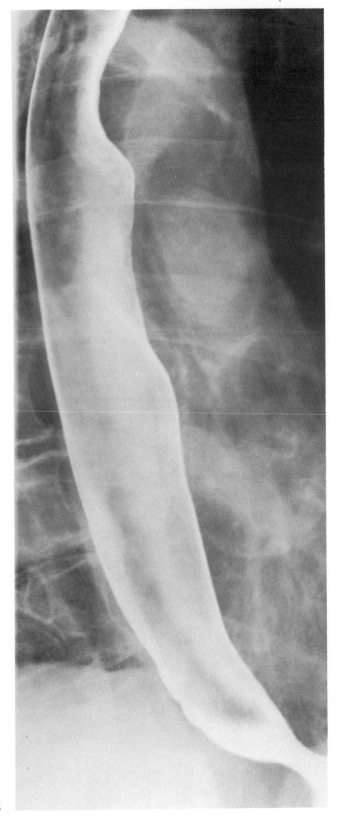

2.10

2.11

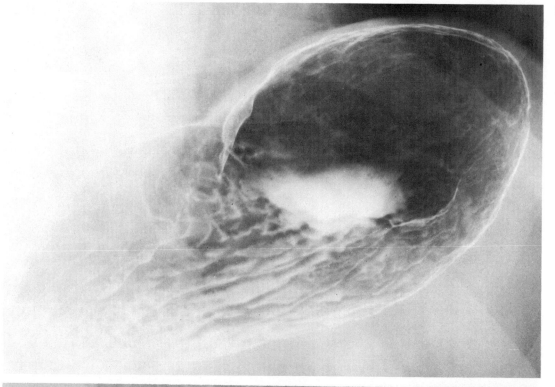

2.12

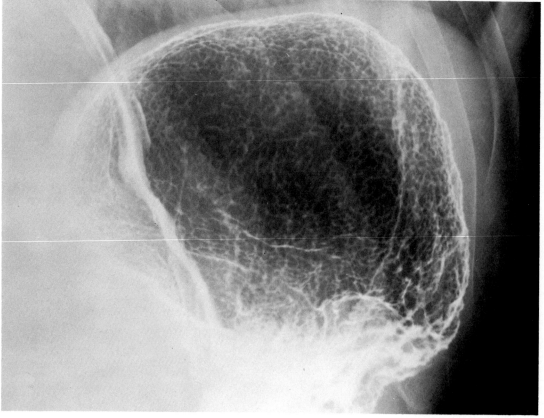

2.13

2.14

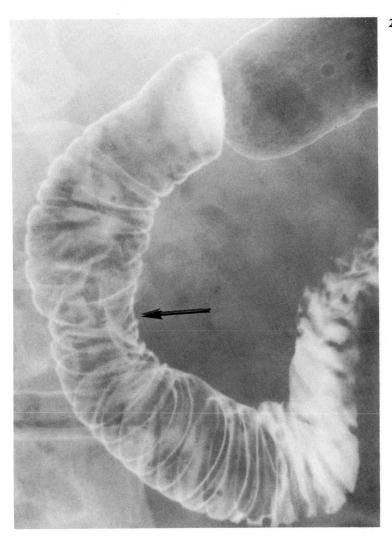

2.15

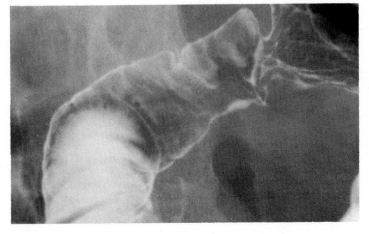

2.12 An example of a *supine oblique* view of the fundus taken with the head of the table tilted up 45°

2.13 A *double-contrast* view of the fundus showing the areae gastricae

2.14 A *double-contrast* view of the duodenal loop; the papilla of Vater can be identified in the second part of the duodenum (arrow)

2.15 A view of the **anastomosis** in a patient with a Billroth I partial gastrectomy

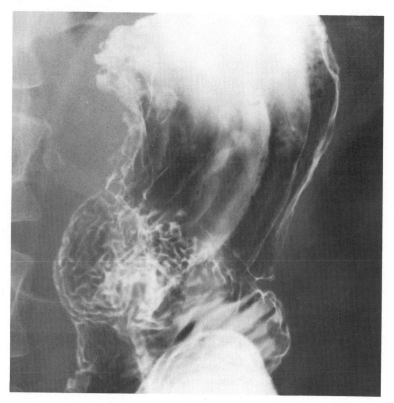

2.16 A *double-contrast* view of a **Billroth II anastomosis**

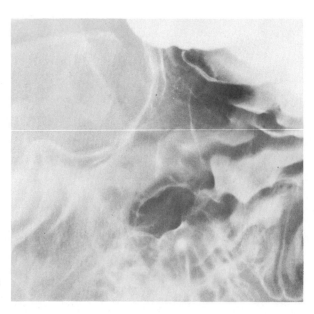

2.17 A **gastroenterostomy anastomosis**
shown on a *double-contrast* view

3 The Oesophagus

The techniques used to examine the oesophagus with barium depend upon the patient's symptoms and the type of lesion suspected. The established methods include the standard barium meal, cineradiography, rapid serial radiography, videotape recording and the special views for demonstrating oesophageal varices. To the list can now be added the double-contrast examination.

Carcinoma of the oesophagus usually presents at a late stage when narrowing of the lumen has occurred. However, some patients develop symptoms at an early stage and a careful study of the oesophagus should be carried out on all patients who present with dysphagia. Double-contrast views of the distended oesophagus facilitate the detection of early oesophageal carcinoma (Suzuki *et al.* 1972; Koehler *et al.* 1976). By obtaining double-contrast views of the oesophagus as part of the double-contrast meal it should be possible to detect a number of carcinomas at an early stage before they become symptomatic.

Benign oesophageal strictures are the other lesions which commonly cause narrowing of the oesophagus and lead to dysphagia. If the narrowing is marked the stricture is best outlined by an opaque barium column. It is important to outline the upper and lower margins of benign strictures so that management can be carefully planned and the results of treatment assessed. Good double-contrast views of benign strictures can be obtained by getting the patient to swallow the barium in the prone position when the fundus of the stomach is well-distended with gas. The gas in the stomach refluxes into the lower oesophagus following the ingestion of barium and outlines the stricture, particularly the lower margin.

Changes in the mucosa of the oesophagus occur in a number of conditions. Moniliasis of the oesophagus is an inflammatory condition with ulceration and pseudomembrane formation and results from infection by the fungus *Candida albicans*. It occurs mostly in patients with debilitating diseases, particularly if they are treated with steroids, antibiotics or immuno-suppressive agents. The classical symptoms are difficulty and pain when swallowing, often associated with persistent retrosternal pain (Holt 1968). The barium-filled oesophagus shows a ragged mucosal outline with pseudopolypoid changes and deep ulceration. Double-contrast views outline the ulcers and their margins particularly well.

Acanthosis nigricans is a cutaneous disorder characterized by papillomatosis, pigmentation and hyperkeratosis. Oesophageal involvement is shown on double-contrast views as fine nodular filling defects throughout the oesophagus, without spiculation (Itai *et al.* 1976, 1977). It is also possible to show leukoplakia of the oesophagus as small superficial protrusions with unsharp margins (Itai *et al.* 1977). Occasionally, herpes oesophagitis may show

changes that resemble moniliasis on double-
contrast views of the oesophagus (Skucas *et al.* 1977).

References

Holt J. M. (1968) *Gut,* **9**, 227

Itai Y., Kogure T., Okuyama Y. & Akiyama H.
(1976) *Br. J. Radiol.,* **49**, 592

Itai Y., Kogure T., Okuyama Y. & Akiyama H.
(1977) *Am. J. Roentgenol.,* **128**, 563

Koehler R. E., Moss A. A. & Margulis A. R. (1976)
Radiology, **119**, 1

Skucas J., Schrank W. W., Meyers P. C. & Lee C. S.
(1977) *Am. J. Roentgenol.,* **128**, 497

Suzuki H., Kobayashi S., Endo M. & Nakayama K.
(1972) *Surgery,* **71**, 99

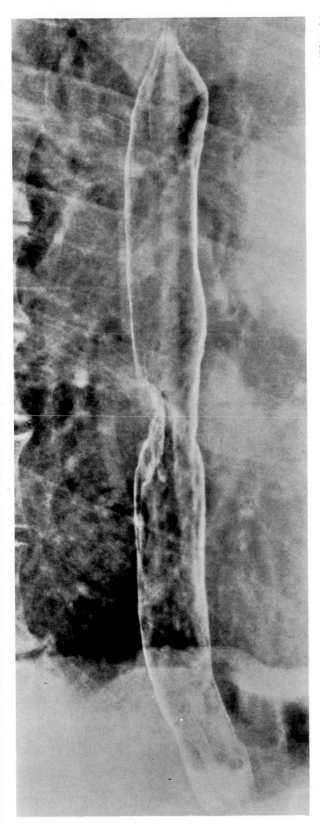

3.1 Carcinoma of the oesophagus A *double-contrast* view shows a carcinoma of the posterior wall of the oesophagus (Courtesy of Dr J. O. Op den Orth)

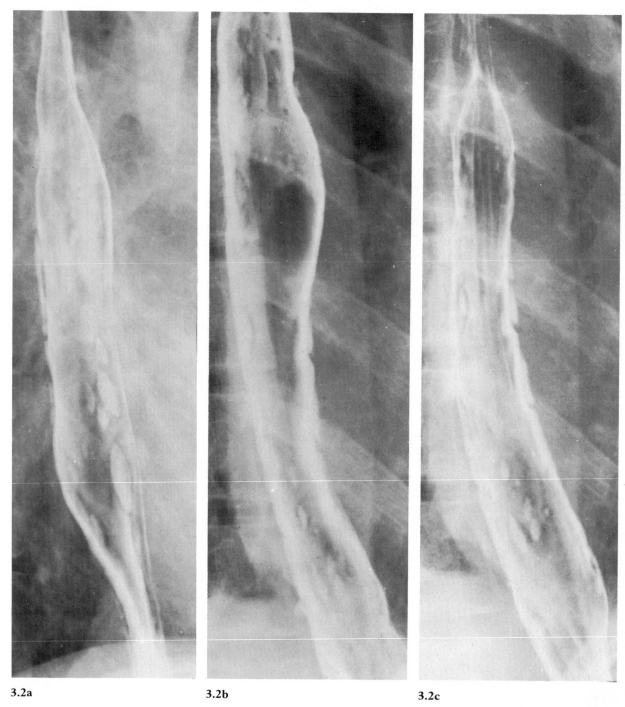

3.2a   3.2b   3.2c

3.2 **Moniliasis of the oesophagus** in a 24-year-old man who developed dysphagia following an emergency colectomy for acute colitis of the entire large intestine

Mucosal ulcers a, b, c of various sizes and shapes are shown in the distal half of the oesophagus. A radiolucent border, presumably due to oedema, surrounds each ulcer. Oesophagoscopy was carried out shortly afterwards, during which white plaques of *Candida albicans* together with punched-out ulcers and oesophagitis were seen. There was an immediate improvement in the patient's symptoms following treatment with nystatin, and a follow-up barium examination showed that the ulcers had healed

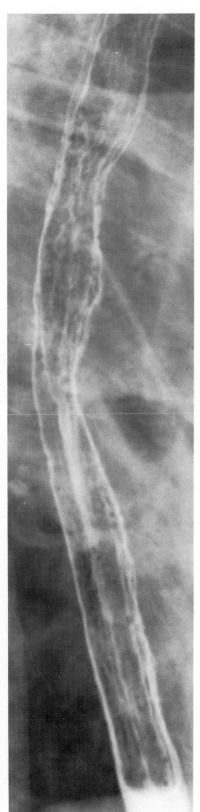

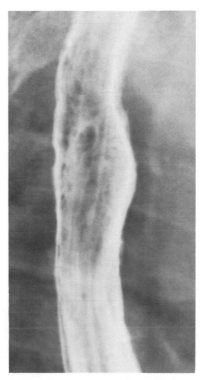

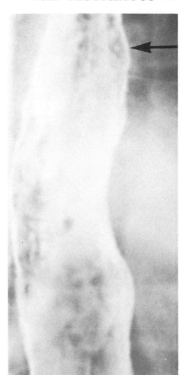

3.3b

3.3c

3.3a

3.3 **Moniliasis of the oesophagus** a Shaggy outline of the mucosa is shown on a *double-contrast* view of the partially distended oesophagus. b, c Films taken when the oesophagus is well-distended show small discrete ulcers with surrounding radiolucent margins (aphthoid ulcers). The radiolucent border is presumably due to oedema

The patient was a 59-year-old female who developed dysphagia while on large doses of steroids for the treatment of systemic lupus erythematosis complicated by arthritis of the hands and pulmonary fibrosis. The throat and palate were red with a white exudate, typical of *Candida albicans*. Immediate relief followed treatment with nystatin

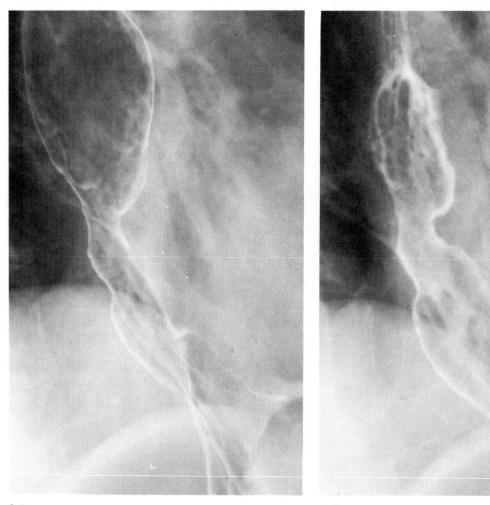

3.4a

3.4b

3.4 Benign oesophageal stricture *Double-contrast* views of the lower oesophagus outline a short benign stricture. Note the rigidity of the stricture while the oesophagus above and below it changes in calibre. a This film shows the upper margin of the stricture; b the lower margin is shown best on this view

3.5

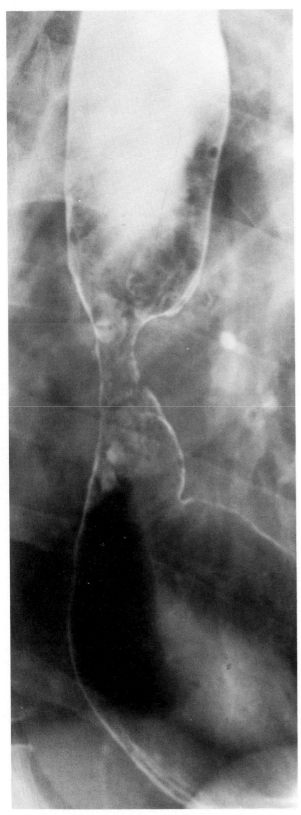

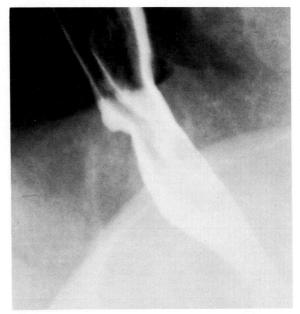

3.6a

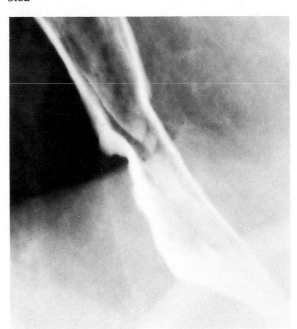

3.6b

3.5 **Benign oesophageal stricture** A hiatal hernia and a benign oesophageal stricture, 5 cm in length, are outlined on a *double-contrast* view of the lower oesophagus and fundus of the stomach. There are a number of ulcers associated with this stricture

3.6 **Oesophageal ulcer and benign stricture** An ulcer associated with a benign stricture is seen

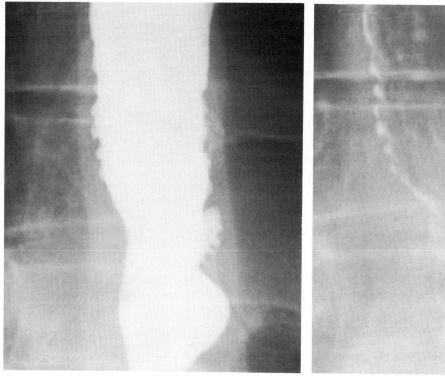

3.7a

3.7b

3.7 Peptic oesophagitis a *Single* and b *double-contrast* views show irregularity and ulceration of the lower oesophagus

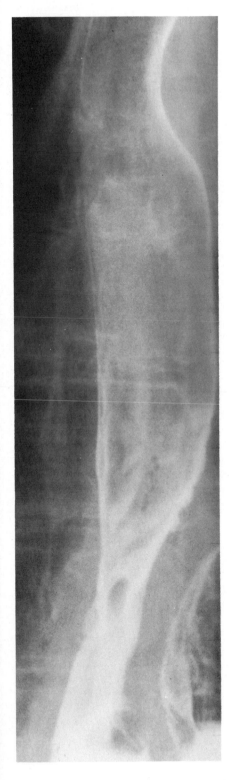

3.8a

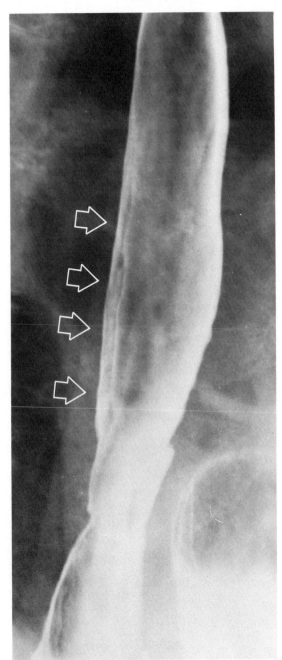

3.8b

3.8 **Hiatal hernia** and **peptic oesophagitis** a, b Ulceration and slight distortion of the lower oesophagus is seen just above the oesophago-gastric junction. A longitudinal ulcer is also present (arrows).

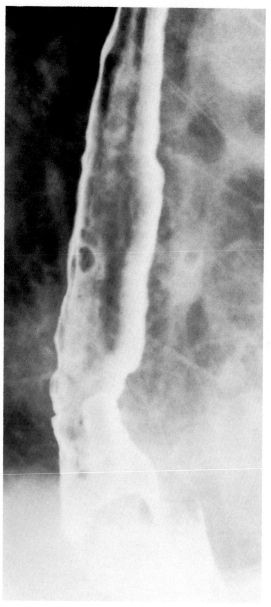

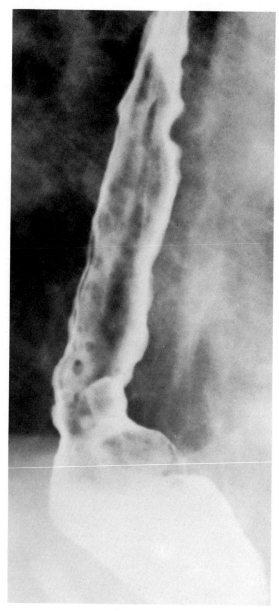

3.9a

3.9b

3.9 **Hiatal hernia** and **peptic oesophagitis** a, b A small hiatal hernia is present and free gastro-oesophageal reflux occurred during the examination. Ulceration and irregularity of the lower oesphagus is seen

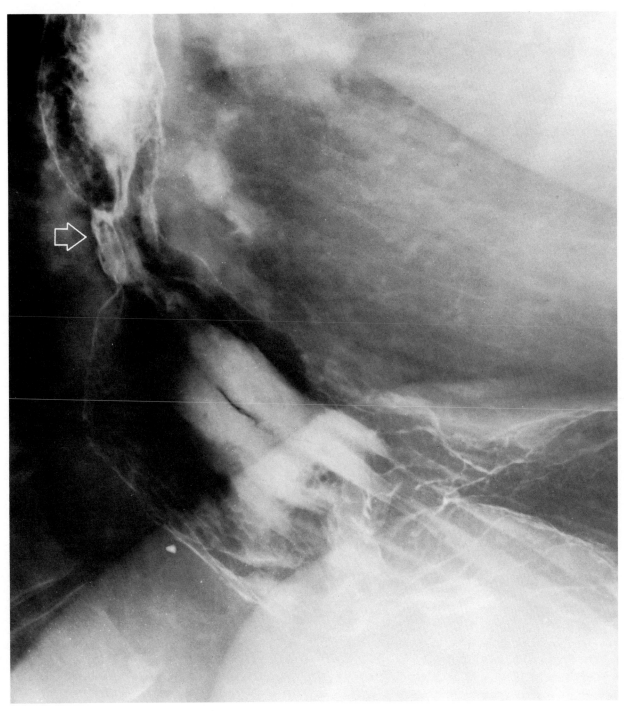

3.10

3.10 **Hiatal hernia** and **peptic ulceration** An oval ulcer crater (arrow) is seen at the oesophago-gastric junction in a patient with a large hiatal hernia. The ulcer was also seen at endoscopy and confirmed at operation

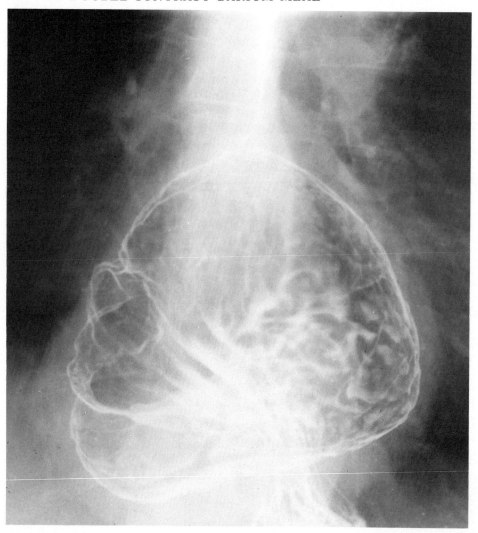

3.11 **Hiatal hernia** A large hiatal hernia outlined during a *double-contrast* study

4 Gastric Ulceration

The stomach and duodenum are the predominant sites of peptic ulceration. A peptic ulcer is a circumscribed lesion involving loss of the full thickness of the mucosa and a variable amount of underlying tissue (Morson & Dawson 1972). Gastric and duodenal ulceration share common pathological features but the difference in incidence, behaviour and pathophysiology of the two conditions strongly suggest that they are separate entities (Crean 1974).

Peptic ulcers may be classified as acute or chronic. It is usually possible to differentiate between acute and chronic peptic ulcers on naked eye appearances, but histological examination is necessary for certainty. The distinction is based on chronicity in the form of fibrosis and cellular infiltration.

In an acute peptic ulcer a little connective tissue is present in the floor of the ulcer or at its margins. When an acute ulcer heals, its floor throws up granulation tissue which in turn is covered by epithelium growing in from the margins (Truelove & Reynell 1972). Some scarring will occur initially when an acute ulcer heals but after a few weeks the site of the original ulcer is difficult or impossible to find.

A chronic peptic ulcer possesses much fibrous tissue and cellular infiltration in its floor and margins. It is slower to heal than an acute ulcer and results in considerable scarring. Healing of a long-established chronic ulcer is a difficult process and the newly formed mucosa is liable to break down into a fresh ulcer.

The incidence of gastric ulcers has decreased considerably, showing a drop of a quarter between 1956 and 1967 (Langman 1974). In the nineteenth century gastric ulceration was extremely common, especially in young women, but it now occurs predominantly in men, in the older age groups and in poorer communities.

Gastric ulcers vary considerably in size; they may be single or multiple, benign or malignant. They occur most commonly along the lesser curve and on the posterior wall of the stomach with very few occurring on the anterior wall (Diagram 4.1). The distribution of gastric ulcers found in double-contrast studies and at endoscopy is similar, with as many occurring in the upper half of the stomach as in the lower half (Stevenson 1977).

The double-contrast barium meal shows gastric ulcers *en face*. This means that the radiographic views show the ulcer crater clearly with detail of the surrounding mucosa. The information thus obtained is similar to that obtained by direct viewing at endoscopy or of the resected specimen. Ulcers may be round, oval or linear and most chronic ulcers have mucosal folds radiating from the edge of the crater. It is easier to differentiate between benign and malignant ulcers when details of the crater and its margins are shown *en face*. The radiating folds are straight and regular in benign cases. Malignancy should be suspected when there is thickening or distortion of the folds at the edge of the ulcer crater, fusion of folds, or

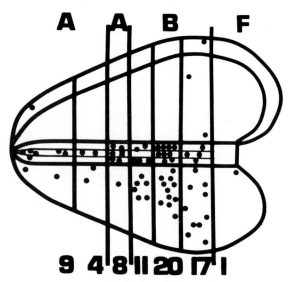

Diag. 4–1 (Stevenson 1977) Diagram to illustrate the position of 70 gastric ulcers found in 56 patients on double-contrast barium meal examination. The drawing depicts a stomach opened from pylorus to cardia along the junction of the posterior wall and greater curve, mucosal surface uppermost with the greater curve at the top of the diagram and the posterior wall at the bottom. Vertical lines divide the proximal and distal antrum, angulus, lower mid- and upper body and fundus

amputation of the fold by an area of induration at the edge of the crater. Ulcers which are shallow with a nodular or uneven pattern in the base and have an ill-defined or irregular outline are usually malignant. Lesions that are suspected of malignancy should be biopsied immediately. Ulcers that may look benign, whether on double-contrast radiographs, at endoscopy or on naked-eye examination, may prove to be malignant. Gastric ulcers, where malignancy has been excluded by histological examination of an adequate number of biopsies, should be followed up with double-contrast radiology to establish that complete healing has taken place.

Superficial mucosal defects which do not penetrate the muscularis mucosa are called erosions, the radiological and endoscopic aspects of which have been the subject of a recent review (Op den Orth & Dekker 1976). When the erosion is surrounded by an elevated zone it is known as a varioliform erosion and multiple gastric varioliform erosions

may be referred to as erosive gastritis. Varioliform erosions are most common in the antrum and many are present on the gastric mucosal folds, and can be diagnosed reliably by using the double-contrast technique.

Recurrent ulceration can be expected in between one and five per cent of patients following surgical treatment for peptic ulceration (Stabile & Passaro 1976). About 95 per cent occur following surgery for duodenal ulcers and are mostly sited at or distal to the anastomosis. A combination of double-contrast radiology and fibre-optic endoscopy is required for complete evaluation of the area around the anastomosis. Billroth I partial gastrectomy anastomosis sites are particularly well shown by the double-contrast technique.

References

Crean G. P. (1974) *Practitioner*, **213**, 27

Langman M. J. S. (1974) Epidemiology of peptic ulcer. In *Gastroenterology*, **1** (Ed. Bockus H. L.) Philadelphia: W. B. Saunders

Morson B. C. & Dawson I. M. P. (1972) *Gastrointestinal Pathology*. Oxford: Blackwell Scientific Publications

Op den Orth J. O. & Dekker W. (1976) *Radiol. Clin. (Basel)*, **45**, 88

Stabile B. E. & Passaro E. (1976) *Gastroenterology*, **70**, 124

Stevenson G. (1977) *Clin. Radiol.*, **28**, 617

Truelove S. C. & Reynell P. C. (1972) *Diseases of the Digestive System*. Oxford: Blackwell Scientific Publications

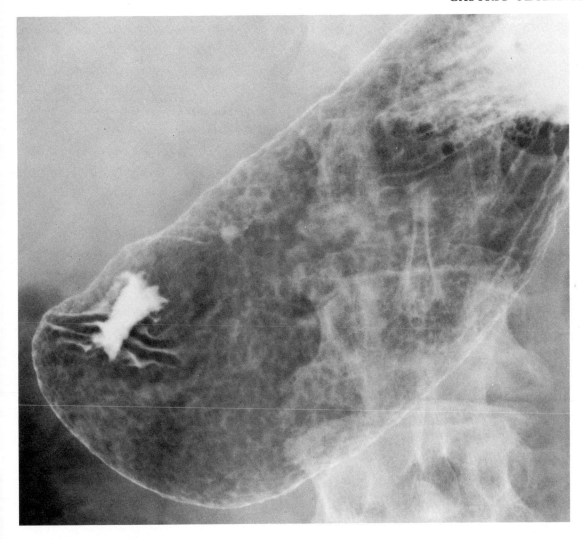

4.1 Gastric ulcer An ulcer crater 5 mm in diameter with short radiating mucosal folds is shown on the posterior wall of the lesser curve aspect of the stomach

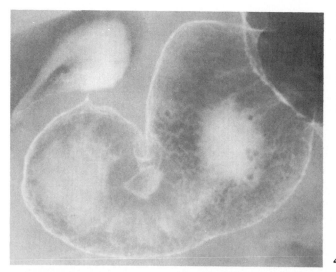

4.2 Hiatal hernia and multiple gastric ulcers

a *Double-contrast* view of the antrum showing a shallow acute ulcer, 8 mm in diameter, with surrounding oedema. b Two further ulcers (arrowed) are seen in a hiatal hernia on *double-contrast* views of the fundus. Biopsies obtained at a subsequent endoscopic examination showed no evidence of malignancy

4.2a

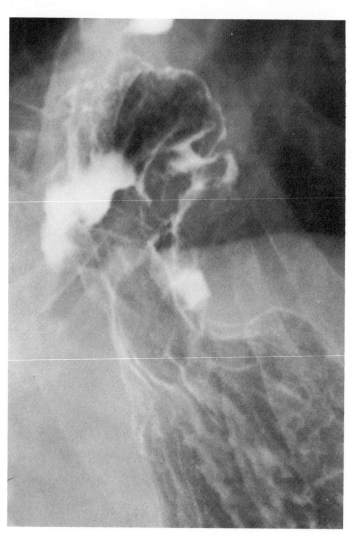

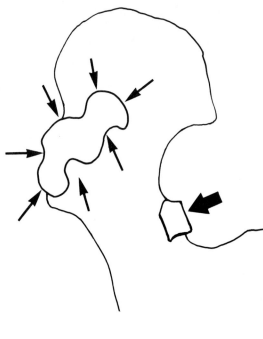

4.2b

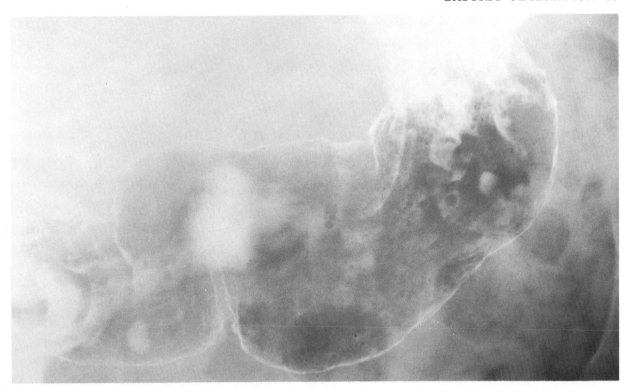

4.3a

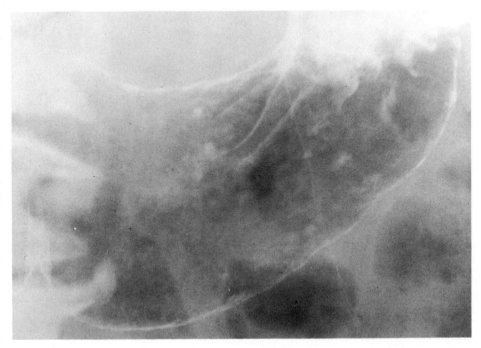

4.3b

4.3 **Multiple acute ulcers** a, b of the body and antrum of the stomach. The findings were confirmed at endoscopy

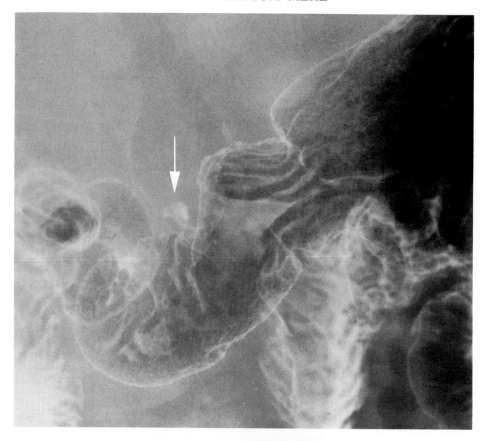

4.4a

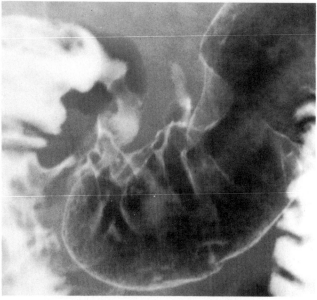

4.4b

4.4 **Antral ulcers and erosions** a, b *Double-contrast* views of the gastric antrum show a lesser curve ulcer, 7 mm in diameter, and multiple tiny ulcers and erosions; these were also seen at endoscopy

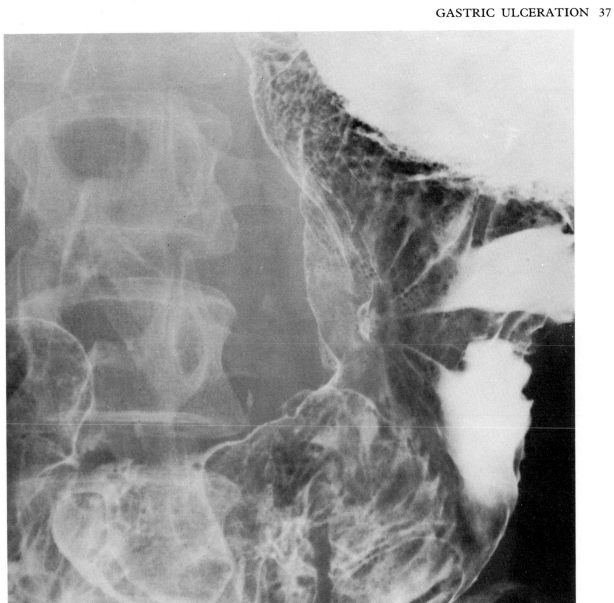

4.5 Benign gastric ulcer Note the straight folds radiating from the edge of the ulcer crater

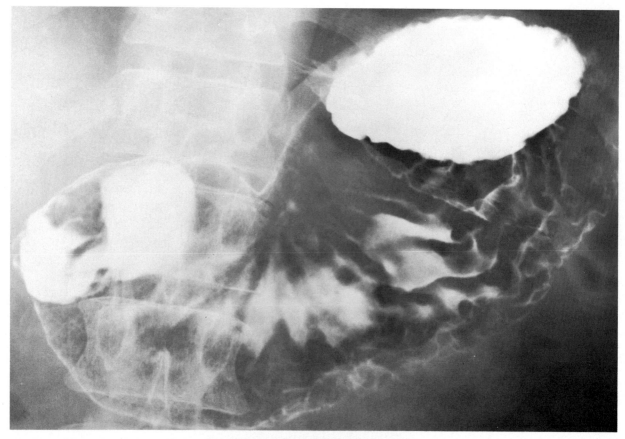

4.6a

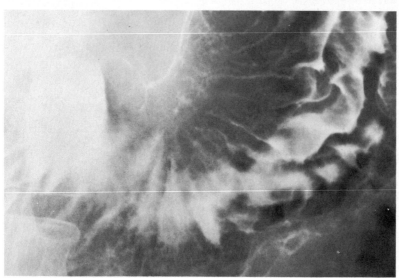

4.6b

4.6 **Chronic gastric ulcer** a, b *Double-contrast* views show
a small ulcer with slightly irregular radiating mucosal folds
that do not extend to the edge of the crater; the irregularity is
probably due to gastritis. The patient had been endoscoped
six months previously when a larger ulcer crater was present.
Biopsies obtained showed no evidence of malignancy

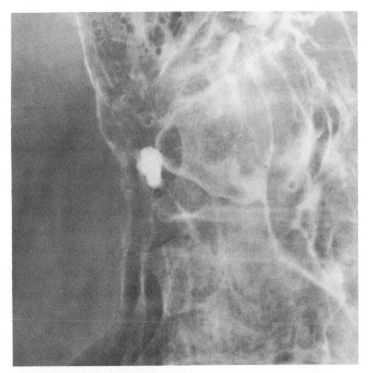

4.7 Chronic gastric ulcer An ulcer crater, 10 mm in diameter, is seen with radiating folds that extend to its edge. The patient, a 78-year-old female with left heart failure, is known to have had a gastric ulcer four years previously

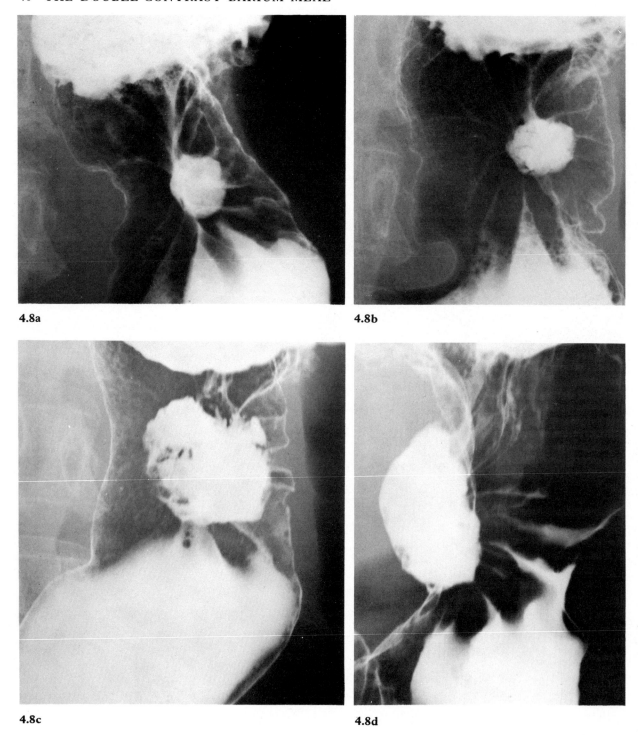

4.8a

4.8b

4.8c

4.8d

4.8 **Chronic benign gastric ulcer** An ulcer crater 2 cm in diameter is seen a, b involving the upper part of the body of the stomach with the mucosal folds extending to the edge of the crater. Two months previously the ulcer had been much larger. Medical treatment was continued but a repeat examination five months later c, d shows that the ulcer has in fact become much larger. A partial gastrectomy was carried out and at operation the ulcer was found to be invading the pancreas. The histological examination revealed no evidence of malignancy

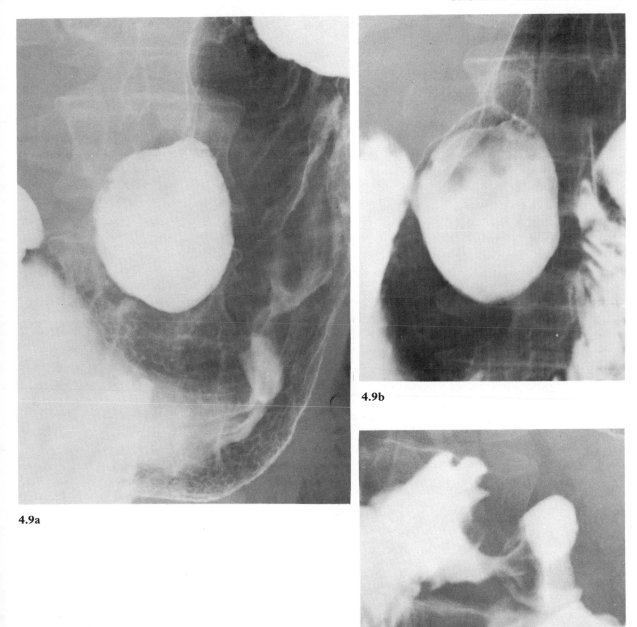

4.9a

4.9b

4.9c

4.9 Large gastric and duodenal ulcers a *Double-contrast* view of the body of the stomach shows a lesser curve gastric ulcer 5 cm in diameter. b A nodular pattern is seen in the base of the ulcer crater; this type of appearance is often seen in the base of gastric ulcers that penetrate the pancreas. c the duodenal cap contains an ulcer 1·5 cm in diameter, which is seen best on a single-contrast view

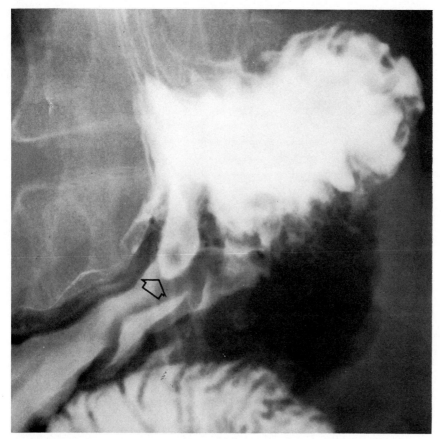

4.10a

4.10b

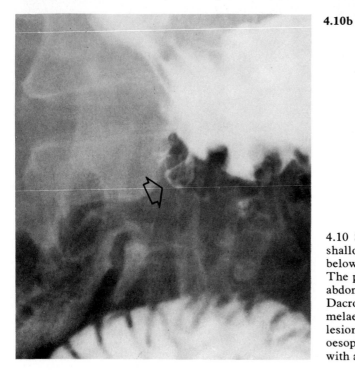

4.10 **Stress ulcer** a, b These views show a
shallow stress ulcer, 7 mm in diameter, just
below the oesophago-gastric junction (arrows).
The patient, a 64-year-old man who had had an
abdominal aortic aneurysm repaired with a
Dacron graft five days previously, developed
melaena. Endoscopy was carried out first, but no
lesion was found. The area adjacent to the
oesophago-gastric junction is difficult to examine
with an end-viewing fibre-optic endoscope

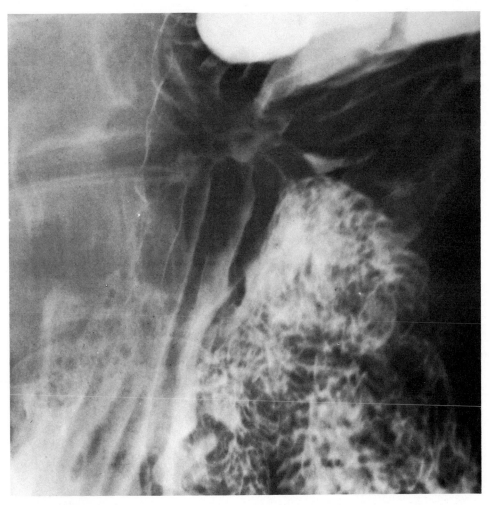

4.11a

4.11b

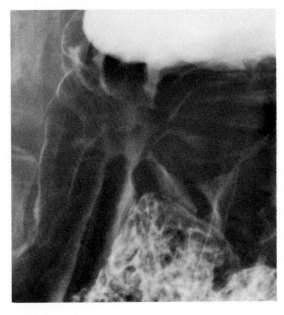

4.11 **Malignant gastric ulcer** *Double-contrast* views a, b demonstrate a shallow ulcer crater with an uneven floor and an irregular ill-defined outline. Some of the converging folds are distorted and fuse while others show widening and clubbing as they reach the edge of the ulcer. Histological examination of the resected specimen showed a poorly differentiated adenocarcinoma, mainly within the mucosa but in some areas spreading into the submucosa and through to the serosa
(Courtesy of Dr J. C. MacLarnon)

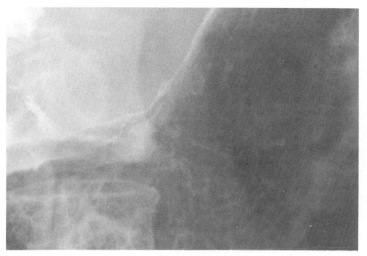

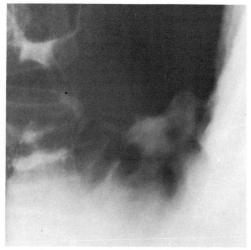

4.12a

4.12b

4.12 Malignant gastric ulcer a *Double-contrast* view showing a poorly defined ulcer crater at the incisura angularis. Uneven and gradual loss of areae gastricae is seen near the ulcer. b A *compression* view shows the irregular outline and a nodular pattern in the base of the crater and around the margin. These appearances indicate that the ulcer is likely to be malignant, but inspection at operation suggested that it was benign. However, on histological examination the ulcer proved to be an adenocarcinoma which was mainly intramucosal but did, in fact, show some extension right out to the serosa

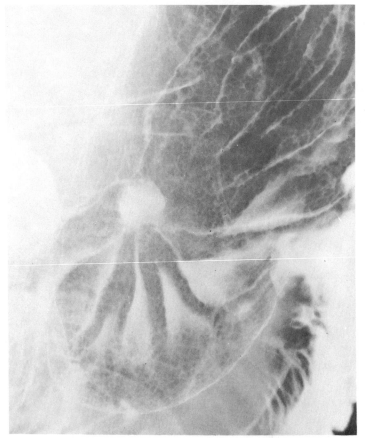

4.13

4.13 Malignant gastric ulcer A *double-contrast* view of the body of the stomach shows an ulcer crater. Mucosal folds extend to the edge of the crater on the inferior aspect but on the superior edge they are interrupted by a featureless area. The areae gastricae pattern is altered near the ulcer, especially where the folds are amputated.
Biopsies obtained at endoscopy showed evidence of malignancy and a gastrectomy was carried out. Histological examination confirmed the ulcer to be an adenocarcinoma extending to the serosa in the base but limited to the mucosa at the edge of the crater

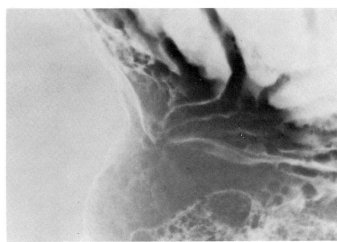

4.14 **Ulcer scar** with radiating mucosal folds

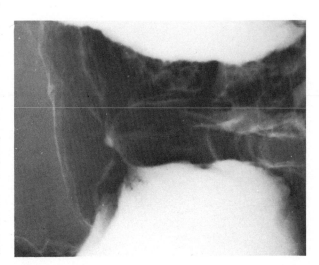

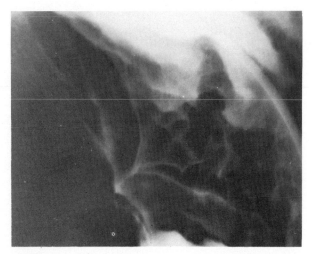

4.15a

4.15b

4.15 **Healing gastric ulcer with radiating folds.** Six weeks previously a benign gastric ulcer was seen at endoscopy

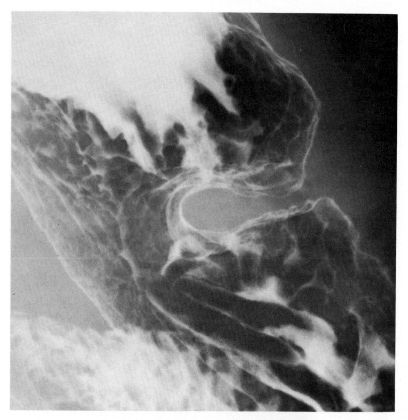

4.16 Ulcer scar A longitudinal ulcer scar with radiating mucosal folds and an 'incisura' of the greater curve is shown where a benign ulcer had been seen at endoscopy three weeks earlier

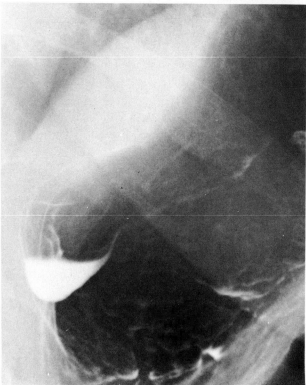

4.17a

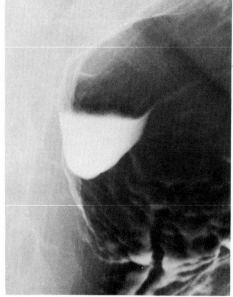

4.17b

4.17 Gastric diverticulum a, b Note the wide neck and the mucosal folds extending into the diverticulum. This is the classic site for gastric diverticula — the posterior aspect of the upper end of the lesser curve

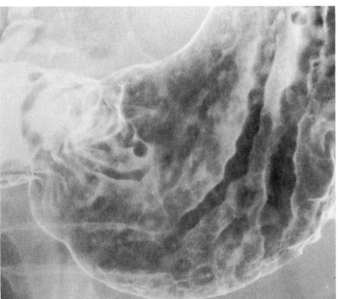

4.18 **Gastric erosions** a, b Multiple small erosions are shown in the body and antrum of the stomach. Note the zone of oedema surrounding each erosion. At endoscopy round oedematous areas 'like polyps with tiny ulcers in the centre' were seen. c An examination carried out six months later shows a reduction in the number of erosions

4.18a

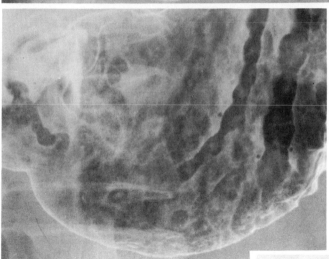

4.18b

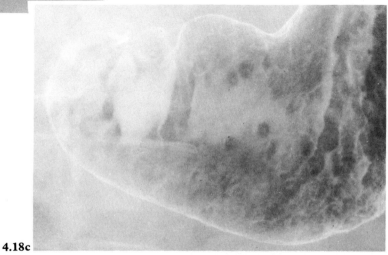

4.18c

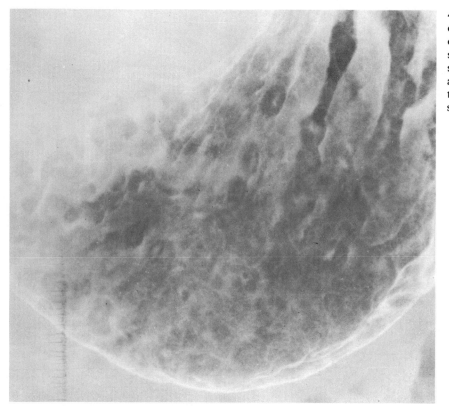

4.19 Gastric erosions Multiple erosions with surrounding oedema are seen in the body and antrum of the stomach; these erosions were also seen at endoscopy

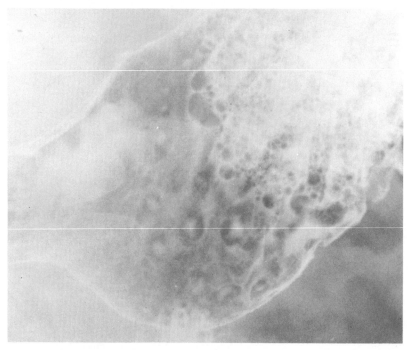

4.20 Gastric erosions A number of large erosions with surrounding oedema are present at the junction of the body and antrum of the stomach

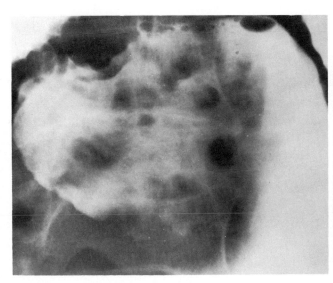

4.21a

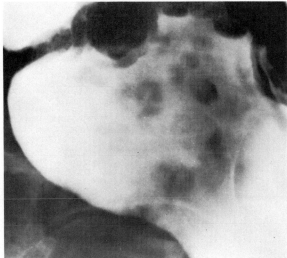

4.21b

4.21 Gastric erosions a, b Multiple small collections of barium with surrounding zones of oedema are shown on *compression* views of the gastric antrum. The patient refused endoscopy: he was treated with cimetidine and the erosions were no longer present when a repeat barium study was carried out three months later

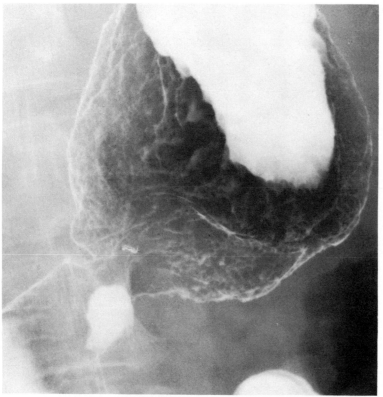

4.22a

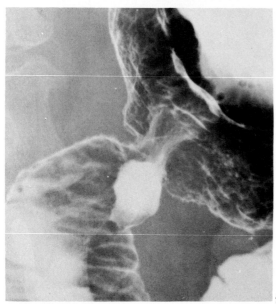

4.22b

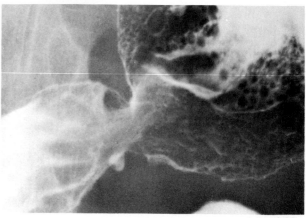

4.22c

4.22 **Anastomotic ulcer** a, b A *double-contrast* examination shows an ulcer crater, 1·5 cm in diameter, at the anastomotic site in a patient with a Billroth I partial gastrectomy who had been admitted with melaena. An opaque barium meal and endoscopy were carried out first but the ulcer was not detected. It was seen when endoscopy was repeated following this examination. c A truncal vagotomy was carried out and a repeat examination three months later shows that the ulcer has almost completely healed

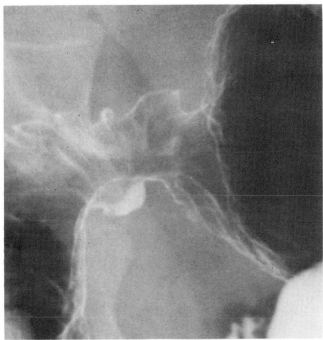

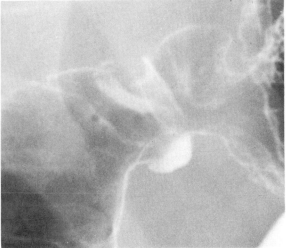

4.23b

4.23a

4.23c

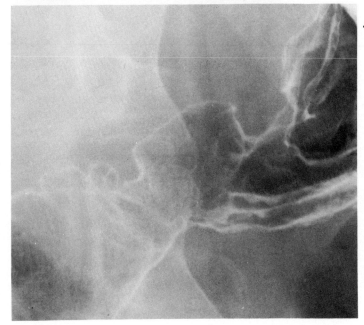

4.23 Recurrent ulcer in a patient with a Billroth I partial gastrectomy A 42-year-old man was admitted with melaena. Endoscopy was carried out but no lesion was found. However, a *double-contrast* study a, b showed an ulcer on the inferior aspect of the duodenum just distal to the site of the anastomosis. A transthoracic truncal vagotomy was carried out and a repeat examination three months later c shows that the ulcer has healed

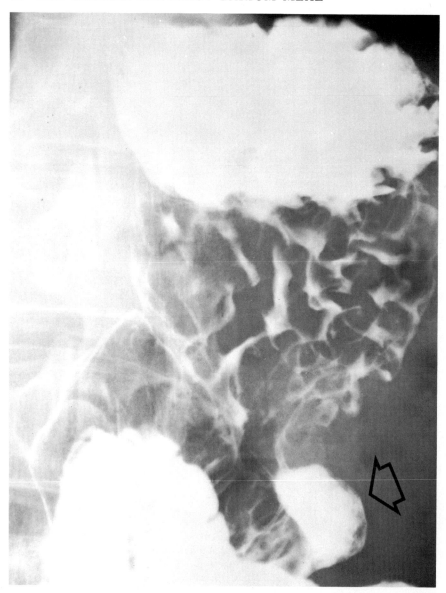

4.24 Recurrent ulceration A large ulcer is seen just distal to the anastomosis site in a patient with a Polya-type partial gastrectomy; it was also seen at endoscopy

Although less frequent than in Japan, gastric cancer is a common cause of death in Europe. The prognosis is generally poor at the time of the diagnosis — the five-year survival rate being 10 per cent.

At the Annual Meetings of the Japanese Gastro-enterological Endoscopic Society in 1962 and of the Japanese Research Society for Gastric Cancer in 1963 early gastric cancer (EGC) was defined as a carcinoma of the stomach whose invasion was limited to the mucosa and submucosa. Neither the size of the carcinoma nor the presence of metastases influences this definition — it is the depth of the infiltration that matters. In 1962 the Japanese Gastroenterological Endoscopic Society proposed a macroscopic classification for EGC that is now being used all over the world (Diagram 5.1).

5 Early Gastric Cancer

J O OP DEN ORTH
W DEKKER

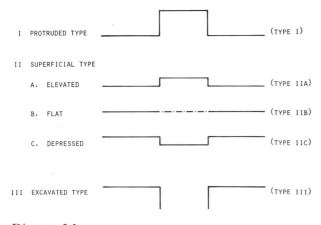

I PROTRUDED TYPE		(TYPE I)
II SUPERFICIAL TYPE		
A. ELEVATED		(TYPE IIA)
B. FLAT		(TYPE IIB)
C. DEPRESSED		(TYPE IIC)
III EXCAVATED TYPE		(TYPE III)

Diagram 5.1

Early gastric cancer has a favourable prognosis. Takasugi *et al.* (1977) analysed the actuarial survival rate of 732 patients with EGC who had had a single lesion operated on at the National Cancer Hospital in Tokyo. The five-year survival rate of all early gastric cancers was 97·7 per cent and the 10-year survival rate 96·4 per cent.

In a general hospital during the three-year period (September 1973–September 1976) 12 cases of early gastric cancer were diagnosed as proved in the resected specimens. During this same period approximately 5,000 radiological gastric examinations were made — always prior to gastroscopy — all but one of which demonstrated definite lesions.

The radiological examination consisted of a standard biphasic contrast gastric series. The term 'biphasic' is used to emphasize that in a routine examination a combination of the conventional barium meal and double-contrast techniques are needed to get a complete visualization of the inner surface of the stomach. Hypotony was obtained in nearly all cases by an intravenous injection of 0·25–0·5 mg of glucagon.

It is our conviction that the part the radiologist plays in diagnosing early gastric cancer is in detecting a potentially malignant lesion. Every gastric ulcer was regarded as such, even without the presence of one of the numerous more-or-less reliable signs of malignancy. Any destruction of the normal mucosal relief showing irregularity, or any polypoid lesion — especially if the diameter was greater than 1 cm or when the surface showed irregularity, was considered a potentially malignant lesion. When there was no absolute contraindication, all patients showing such lesions were endoscoped.

In order to achieve a very high degree of accuracy many (more than 10) endoscopically-directed biopsy specimens were taken after painstaking endoscopic inspection of the gastric mucosa. If all biopsy specimens were negative in spite of radiological and endoscopic investigations, a second gastroscopy for the purpose of taking even more biopsies was performed. Finally, the depth of infiltration was determined in the resected specimen by the pathologist.

References

Dekker W. & Op den Orth J. O. (1977) *Radiol. Clin. (Basel)*, **46**, 115

Takasugi T. *et al.* (1977) *Stomach & Intest.* **12**, 933

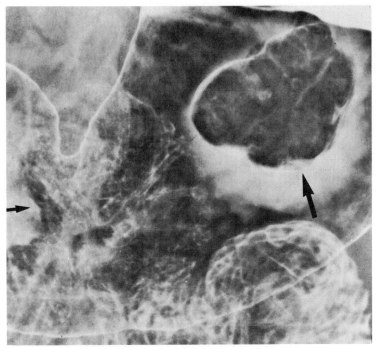

5.1 **Early gastric cancer** in a 75-year-old woman *Double-contrast* picture in the supine position. The large arrow points to a fairly large irregular polypoid lesion on the posterior wall of the corpus, and the small arrow to a garland-like lesion on the posterior wall of the angulus. Both lesions are highly suspicious of malignancy. Gastrobiopsy proved adenocarcinoma. The resected specimen showed that both carcinomas were EGC confined to the submucosa. The large lesion can be classified as Type I; the small one as Type IIa

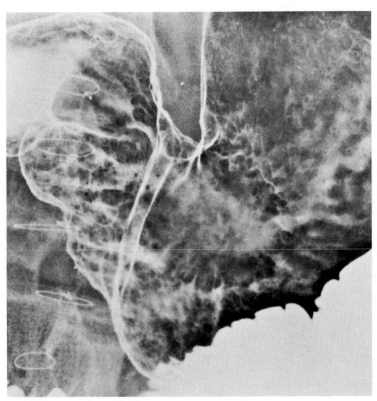

5.2 **Early gastric cancer** in a man of 81 years of age. *Double-contrast* study in the supine position. On the posterior wall of the antrum, near the angulus, there is a rather flat lesion, the normal relief having been destroyed. This picture is highly suspicious of EGC Type II. Gastrobiopsy proved adenocarcinoma. In the resected specimen the diagnosis of EGC was proved and the adenocarcinoma was confined to the mucosa

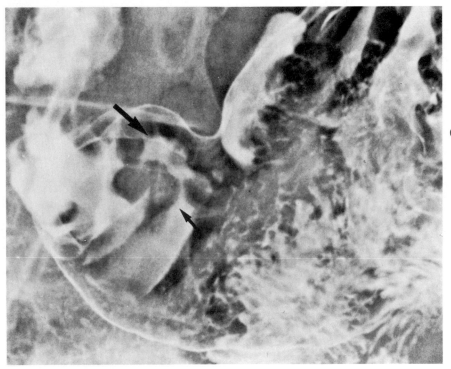

5.3 **Early gastric cancer** in a 43-year-old woman. *Double-contrast* study in the supine position. The large arrow points to an irregular niche, and the small arrow to swollen folds surrounding the niche. This picture is highly suspicious of malignancy (the shadow superimposed on the minor curvature is caused by a duodenal diverticulum). Gastrobiopsy proved adenocarcinoma. The resected specimen showed that the carcinoma was confined to the submucosa, proving the diagnosis of EGC Type III

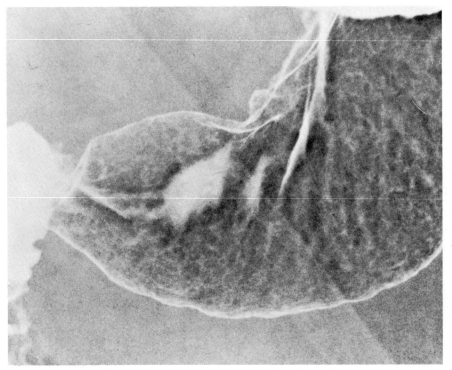

5.4 **Early gastric cancer** in a man of 64 years of age. *Double-contrast* study in the supine position. In the angulus there is an elevated lesion with two niches. The radiological picture is highly suspicious of malignancy, and gastrobiopsy showed adenocarcinoma. In the resected specimen the carcinoma was confined to the mucosa. We may call this EGC of a mixed type

The commonest benign tumours of the stomach are leiomyomas and adenomatous polyps. The first radiological diagnosis of a gastric polyp was made by Heinz in 1911 (Heinz 1912), and Schindler in 1922 was the first to visualize a gastric polyp through a gastroscope. However, it is only since the advent of double-contrast radiology and fibre-optic endoscopy that it has become possible reliably to detect small gastric polyps.

On double-contrast views of the stomach, polyps appear as filling defects with a sharply-defined outer border which is often slightly irregular. The stalks of pedunculated polyps may be visible. Gas bubbles are sometimes confusing as they can look like polyps, but they do not have the sharply-defined border or the slightly irregular outline. Gas bubbles can also collect around polyps and obscure them. If there is doubt about the presence of gastric polyps a number of films of a suspected lesion should be taken and the area washed with barium between each exposure. Polyps in the body and antrum of the stomach can also be demonstrated on compression views.

Leiomyomas are the most common benign tumours of the stomach; the autopsy incidence in one series was as high as 16 per cent (McNeer & Pack 1967). The majority of leiomyomas are small and usually asymptomatic. Haematemesis and melaena occur more commonly than with other gastric tumours, and bleeding tends to be repetitive and copious.

Small adenomatous polyps are almost always benign but some of the larger ones may show changes of epithelial atypia, which is considered on morphological appearances to be carcinoma *in situ* (Monaco *et al.* 1962). While there is no evidence that these polyps become invasive, it is important to note that sessile polypoid tumours larger than 2 cm in diameter may represent frank polypoid carcinomata. There is a high incidence of malignancy when polyps are multiple. Adenomatous polyps are usually symptomless but patients may complain of upper abdominal discomfort. They may bleed which in some patients results in iron deficiency anaemia; they may also be associated with pernicious anaemia. Very occasionally, large pedunculated polyps may prolapse into the duodenum and produce gastric obstruction.

There are two uncommon conditions, juvenile polyposis and the Cronkhite-Canada syndrome, in which polyps are found in the stomach. The histological appearances of the polyps found in both these conditions are somewhat similar and the polyps are considered to have little or no malignant potential. Alopecia, nail dystrophy and hyperpigmentation of the skin, associated with polyps of the stomach and intestines are the features of the Cronkhite–Canada syndrome (Cronkhite & Canada 1955). Other benign polypoid lesions, which are rare, include

6 Benign Neoplasms of the Stomach

D J NOLAN
B S ANAND

lipomas, angiomas, glomus tumours and carcinoid tumours.

Biopsies obtained at gastroscopy fail to give a histological diagnosis of the type of polyp. The biopsy specimens so obtained normally only show the nature of the mucosa covering the polyp. For a full histological diagnosis it is necessary to remove one or more of the polyps by snaring them at gastroscopy, the technique being similar to that used for removing colonic polyps.

References

Cronkhite L. W. Jr & Canada W. J. (1955) *New Engl. J. Med.,* **252,** 1011

Heinz (1912) Korresp. *-Bl. schweiz Ärz.,* **42,** 354, quoted by Spriggs E. I. & Marxer O. A. (1943) *Quart. J. Med.,* **36,** 1

McNeer G. & Pack G. T. (1967) *Neoplasms of the Stomach.* Philadelphia: J. B. Lippincott

Monaco A. P., Roth S. I., Castleman B. & Welch C. E. (1962) *Cancer,* **15,** 456

Schindler R. (1922) *Münch. med. Wschr.,* **69,** 535

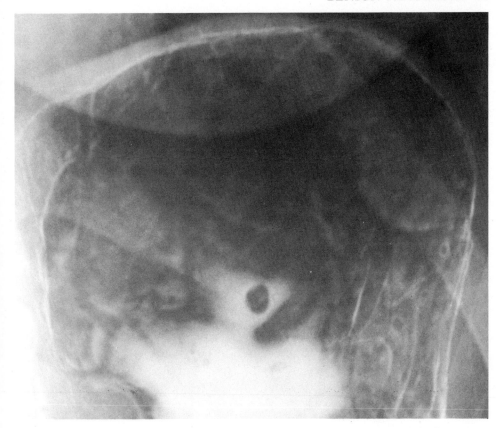

6.1a

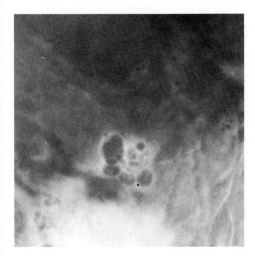

6.1b

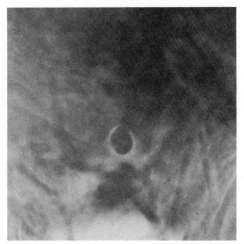

6.1c

6.1 A **solitary polyp**, 7 mm in diameter, is shown at the junction of the body and fundus of the stomach. In a it is surrounded by a thin layer of barium; b gas bubbles are caught at the margin of the polyp; c the barium and gas bubbles have drained away and the sharply-defined outer margin of the polyp is clearly seen. Biopsies obtained at endoscopy showed normal gastric mucosa

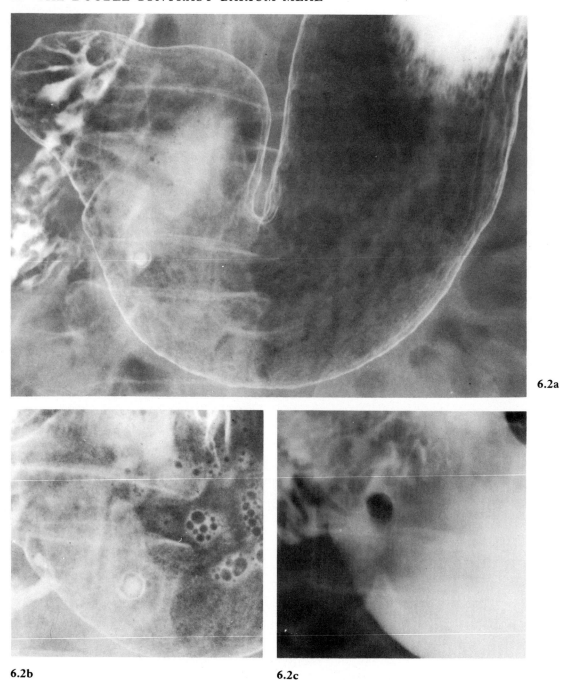

6.2a

6.2b

6.2c

6.2 *Double-contrast* views a, b demonstrate an **anterior wall polyp** near the greater curve aspect of the gastric antrum, with well-defined slightly irregular margins. The dense collection of barium at the centre represents a drop of barium hanging from the polyp, the 'stalactite sign'. c A *compression* view

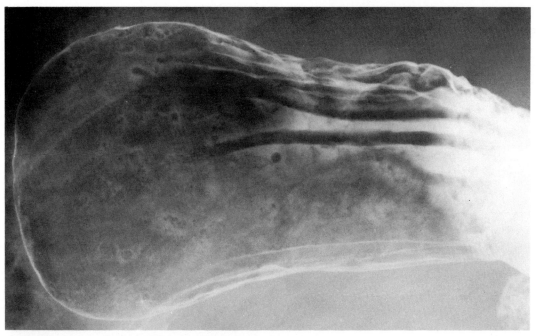

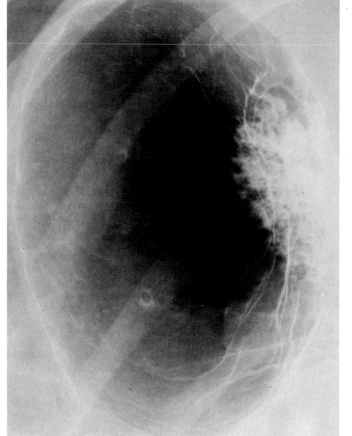

6.3 A *double-contrast* view of the fundus of the stomach shows **two small polyps**, each about 3 mm in diameter; these were also seen at endoscopy

6.4 **Multiple small polyps** in the fundus and body of the stomach. Histological examination of biopsies obtained from the polyps and the adjacent stomach wall showed normal gastric mucosa

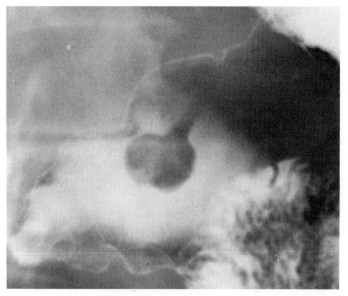

6.5a

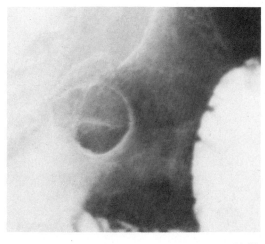

6.5b

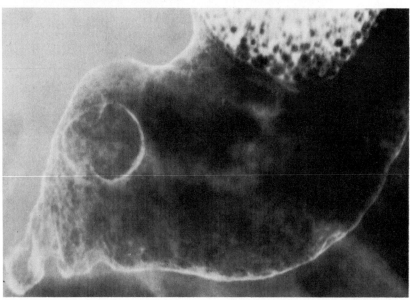

6.5c

6.5 **Large pedunculated antral polyp** a is shown surrounded by a thin layer of barium. b, c Mucosal relief views show the sharply-defined, slightly irregular margin of the polyp. Gastroscopy was not carried out because the patient, a 79-year-old man, was in severe congestive heart failure

FACING PAGE
6.6 **Multiple gastric polyps** a, b, c *Double-contrast* views show a large number of sessile and pedunculated polyps in the body of the stomach with relative sparing of the fundus and antrum. (*continued overleaf*)

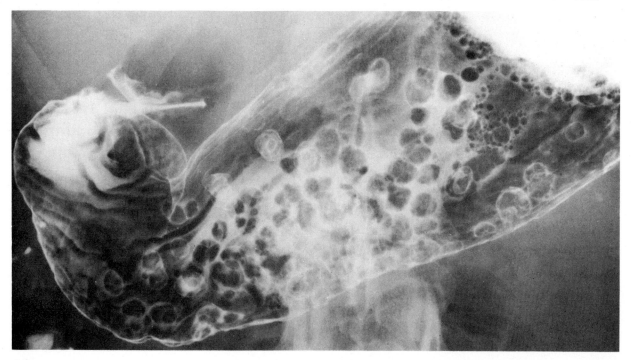

6.6a

6.6b

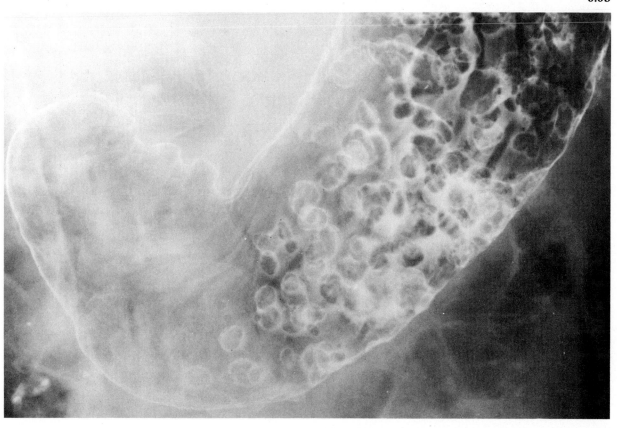

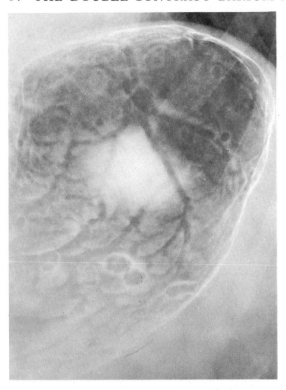

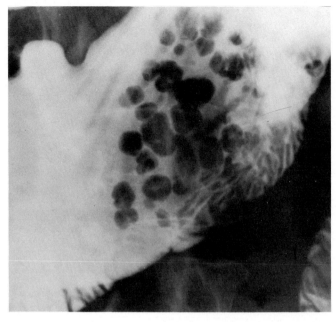

6.6d

6.6c

6.6 (*continued*) d view of the polyps obtained with *compression.* Barium examination of the small and large intestine failed to reveal any further polyps.

Two polyps were removed at gastroscopy and histological examination showed that they were of the type found in juvenile polyposis and the Cronkhite-Canada syndrome. The patient, a 49-year-old female, had no clinical manifestations of the Cronkhite-Canada syndrome

FACING PAGE

6.7 Multiple gastric polyps a Prone *single-contrast* view of the anterior wall of the stomach shows polyps in the body of the stomach as filling defects with well-defined margins. b *Double-contrast* view showing the polyps. No polyps were detected in the small or large intestine. Histological examination of two polyps removed at endoscopy showed that they were of the type found in juvenile polyposis and the Cronkhite-Canada syndrome; the patient had no clinical manifestations of the Cronkhite-Canada syndrome

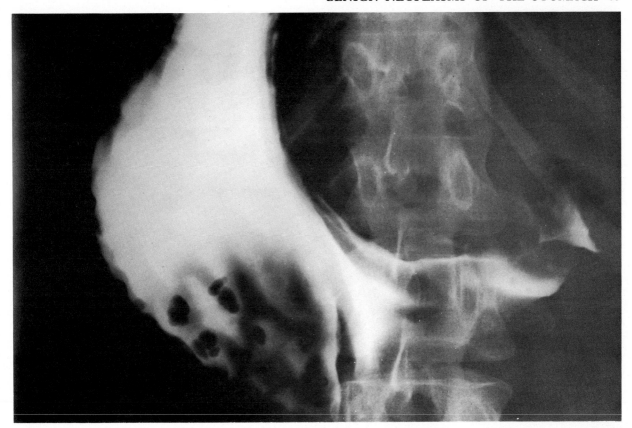

6.7a

6.7b

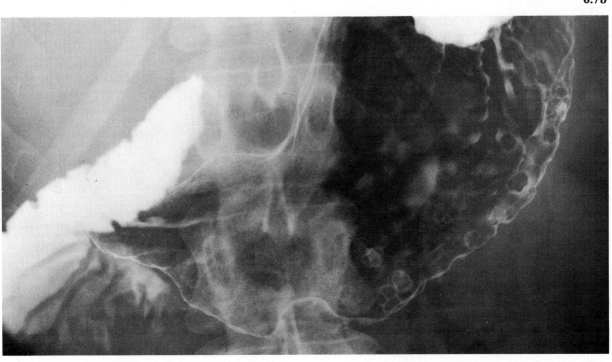

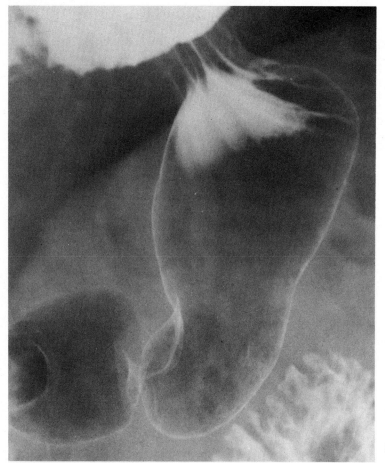

6.8a

6.8b

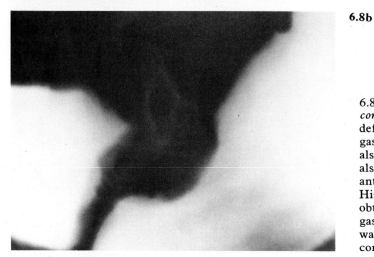

6.8 **Leiomyoma of the stomach** *Double-contrast* view a shows a shallow filling defect on the lesser curve aspect of the gastric antrum. A large hiatal hernia is also present. b The filling defect was also shown on *compression* views of the antrum.

Histological examination of specimens obtained at endoscopy showed normal gastric mucosa. A partial gastrectomy was carried out and the diagnosis confirmed

6.9 Carcinoid tumour of the stomach a, b, c
A tumour, 2 cm in diameter with central ulceration, is shown in the upper part of the body of the stomach. Gastroscopy was carried out and biopsies obtained. Histological examination of the specimens suggested that the tumour might be malignant. The patient was operated on and examination of a frozen section indicated that the lesion was a carcinoid tumour and this was confirmed after the tumour was resected

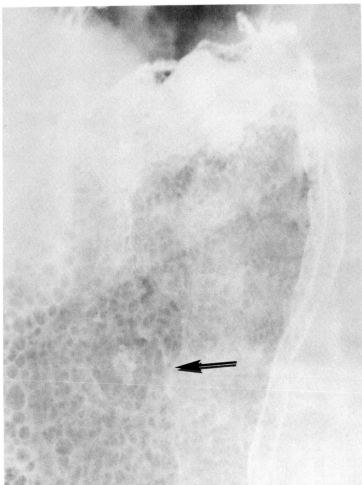

6.9a

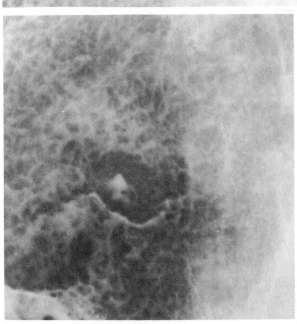

.9b

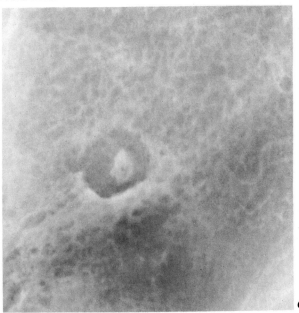

6.9c

7 The Duodenum

Peptic ulceration is the most commonly encountered disease of the duodenum and it usually involves the duodenal cap. Duodenal ulceration tends to be chronic and to recur. It is more common in males with the ratio changing slightly depending on age. There is an incidence of 2 per cent in males compared to 0·5 per cent in females at about 30 years of age, but between 40 and 45 years of age 3 per cent of males and 1 per cent of females will have an active duodenal ulcer during each year (Walker 1973). Ulceration of the duodenum distal to the cap, usually called postbulbar ulceration, is uncommon. Postbulbar ulceration may have a variety of causes such as benign peptic ulceration, the Zollinger-Ellison syndrome, primary carcinoma of the duodenum or the extension into the duodenum of a malignant process in an adjacent organ. The chief complications of duodenal ulceration are bleeding, perforation, and obstruction which, although sited in the duodenum, is often mistakenly called pyloric stenosis.

A double-contrast barium meal examination which includes a view of the cap in the prone position is an accurate method for detecting duodenal ulcers. Ulcer craters show up as sharply-defined, constant collections of barium on double-contrast views; anterior wall ulcers may show as ring shadows when the barium drops from the centre of the crater. The duodenal cap is often deformed as a result of chronic or previous ulceration.

Benign lesions that may appear as filling defects in the duodenum include Brunner's gland adenomas, adenomatous or hamartomatous polyps, ectopic pancreatic tissue, carcinoid tumours and leiomyomas.

Duodenal diverticula are seen in about five per cent of barium studies and are acquired lesions caused by the mucosal and submucosal layers herniating through a muscular defect (Eaton & Ferrucci 1973); the concave border of the descending duodenum is the most common site. Complications are rare but duodenal diverticula may perforate, bleed, or become infected. Cholangitis or pancreatitis may result from the aberrant insertion of the common bile or pancreatic ducts into a duodenal diverticulum (Costopoulos & Miller 1967; Rose 1975).

Until recently duodenal involvement was thought to occur in about four per cent of patients with Crohn's disease of the ileum, jejunum or colon (Fielding *et al.* 1970). However, Stevenson (1978) has found that when double-contrast techniques were used abnormalities suggestive of gastro-duodenal Crohn's disease were shown in 21 per cent of patients with ileal and/or colonic Crohn's disease. Duodenal Crohn's disease is seen as an isolated segment of disease or in continuity with gastric or jejunal Crohn's disease. The radiological appearances of Crohn's disease of the duodenum are similar to those seen in the more distal small intestine (Legge *et al.* 1970). Mucosal thickening and deformity appear in the early stages while mucosal ulceration is seen when the condition is well-established. A varying degree of narrowing of the involved segment may be seen and if the stenosis is marked the more proximal duodenum or stomach may be dilated. When the stomach and duodenum are each involved the normal anatomical landmarks of the antrum, pylorus and duodenal cap are lost and are replaced by a tubular or tapered narrowing. This appearance has been termed the 'pseudo-post-Billroth I' (Nelson 1969). The normal segments and mucosal lesions are seen best on double-contrast views; however, the narrowed segments are best demonstrated by the single-contrast barium column.

Primary carcinoma of the duodenum is uncommon but carcinoma of the head of the pancreas may distort and displace the duodenum. Enlargement of the head of the pancreas due to acute or chronic pancreatitis may also cause changes in the duodenal loop. A mass in the head of the pancreas may displace or cause widening of the duodenal loop or cause a concave pressure defect which, at duodenography, shows as a double contour on the concave border of the duodenum. Other signs of pancreatic enlargement include distortion of the mucosal folds on the concave border of the duodenum and the reversed '3' sign of Frostberg (1938). Malignant tumours in other organs such as the colon, gallbladder or kidney may cause changes in the duodenal loop.

References

Costopoulos L. B. & Miller J. D. R. (1967) *Radiology*, **89**, 256

Eaton, S. B. & Ferrucci J. T. (1973) *Radiology of the Pancreas and Duodenum.* Philadelphia: W. B. Saunders

Fielding J. F., Toye D. K. M., Beton D. C. & Cooke W. T. (1970) *Gut*, **11**, 1001

Frostberg N. (1938) *Acta Radiol.*, **19**, 164

Legge D. A., Carlson H. C. & Judd E. S. (1970) *Am. J. Roentgenol.*, **110**, 355

Nelson S. W. (1969) *Am. J. Roentgenol.*, **107**, 86

Rose P. G. (1975) *Clin. Radiol.*, **26**, 121

Stevenson G. W. (1978) *Gut*, **19**, 962

Walker C. O. (1973) *Chronic Duodenal Ulcer in Gastrointestinal Disease.* (Ed. Sleisenger M. H. & Fordtran J. S.) Philadelphia: W. B. Saunders

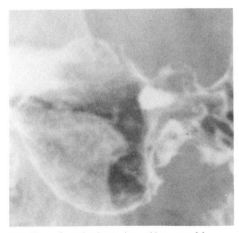

7.1 **Duodenal ulcer** in a 61-year-old man admitted to hospital with melaena. An ulcer is shown in the base of a slightly deformed duodenal cap; it was also seen at endoscopy

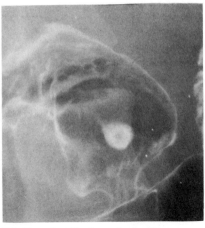

7.2 **Duodenal ulcer** A *double-contrast* view; the cap is not deformed

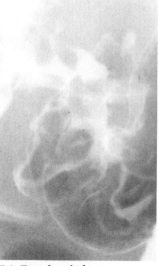

7.3 **Duodenal ulcer**
A deformed duodenal cap containing a medium-sized ulcer crater is shown in a patient who presented with haematemesis and melaena. The findings were confirmed at operation

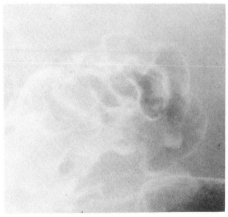

7.4 **Duodenal ulcer**
A *double-contrast* view shows an ulcer crater with radiating mucosal folds in the base of the duodenal cap. This 72-year-old male patient presented with a one-week history of indigestion and melaena

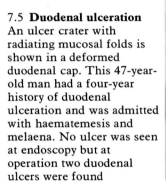

7.5 **Duodenal ulceration**
An ulcer crater with radiating mucosal folds is shown in a deformed duodenal cap. This 47-year-old man had a four-year history of duodenal ulceration and was admitted with haematemesis and melaena. No ulcer was seen at endoscopy but at operation two duodenal ulcers were found

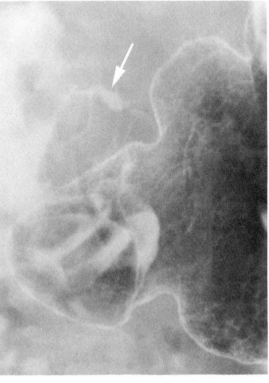

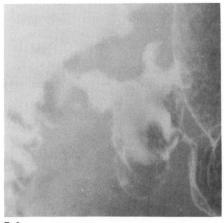

7.6a

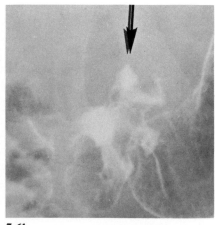

7.6b

7.6 **Duodenal ulceration**
a, b *Double-contrast* views of
the duodenal cap show that
it is grossly deformed. Two
ulcer craters are seen: the
larger is 1 cm in diameter
and irregular in outline,
while the second ulcer can
be seen in the superior part
of the duodenal cap (arrow)

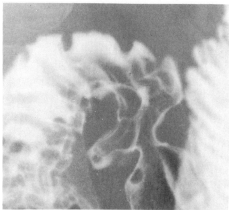

7.7a

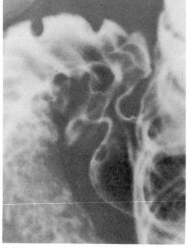

7.7b

7.7 **Duodenal ulcer** a, b
A small ulcer crater with
radiating mucosal folds is
shown on *double-contrast*
views of the duodenal cap.
This ulcer was also seen at
endoscopy

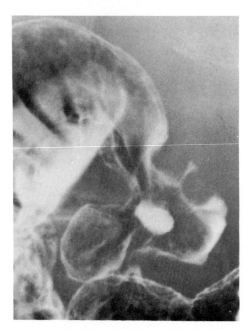

7.8 **Duodenal ulcer** The duodenal cap is deformed and
contains a moderately-sized oval ulcer crater. The patient
presented to his general practitioner complaining of
dyspepsia

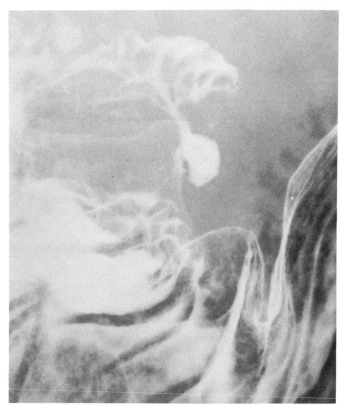

7.9 Duodenal ulceration with gross deformity of the duodenal cap. The duodenal cap is considerably deformed and narrowed with an ulcer crater, 1 cm in diameter, projecting posteriorly. The findings were confirmed at operation

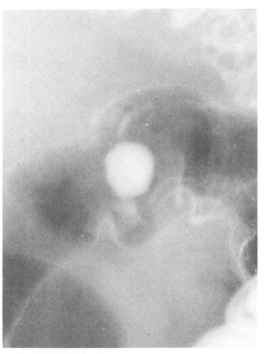

7.10 Duodenal ulcer This patient, who had had a vagotomy and pyloroplasty 10 years previously, was admitted with melaena. Endoscopy was carried out shortly after admission. During the procedure a large amount of blood was present in the stomach and bright red blood was found to be refluxing from the duodenum but no intrinsic lesion of the duodenal cap was seen. A *double-contrast* barium study carried out four days later shows a round ulcer crater, 1·2 cm in diameter, in the duodenal cap (Courtesy of Dr J. C. MacLarnon)

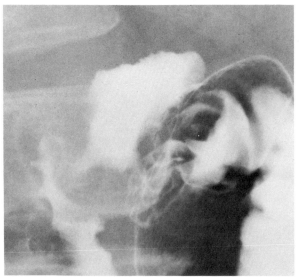

7.11a

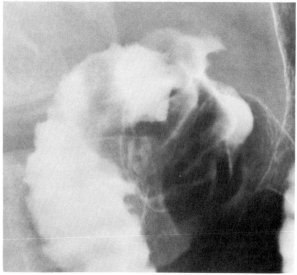

7.11b

7.11 Giant duodenal ulcer a, b *Double-contrast* views show a large ulcer crater in the superior aspect of the duodenal cap of a patient who was admitted because of severe abdominal pain. A *single-contrast* examination three weeks earlier had failed to show the ulcer.
Following the diagnosis, medical treatment was prescribed as the patient also had psychiatric problems. However, he did not respond adequately and was eventually operated on 17 months later, when anterior duodenal adhesions were found with an ulcer crater in the antero-superior aspect of the duodenal cap

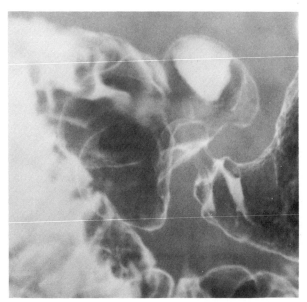

7.12 Deformed duodenal cap due to previous ulceration. A *double-contrast* view of the duodenal cap shows that it is deformed but no ulcer crater can be identified. The gastric mucosa is also prolapsed at the base. The findings at endoscopy were similar

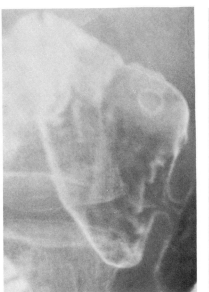

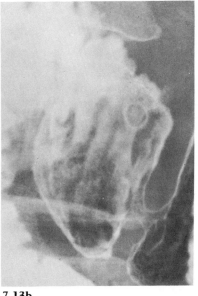

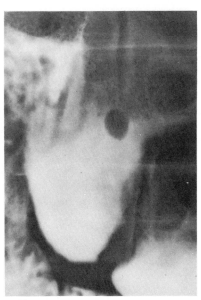

7.13a   **7.13b**   **7.13c**

7.13 Duodenal polyp a, b *Double-contrast* views of the duodenal cap show a round polyp 6 mm in diameter. c The polyp is also seen when the duodenal cap is filled with barium. No other lesion was seen at the barium examination and the patient, a 70-year-old man, was not investigated further

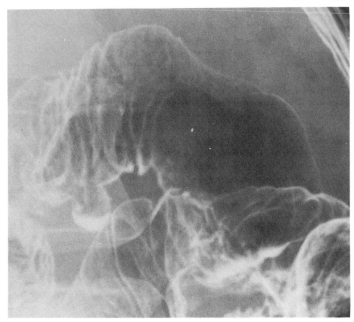

7.14 Duodenal diverticulum A small diverticulum, containing a fluid level of barium, is seen at the proximal end of the descending duodenum

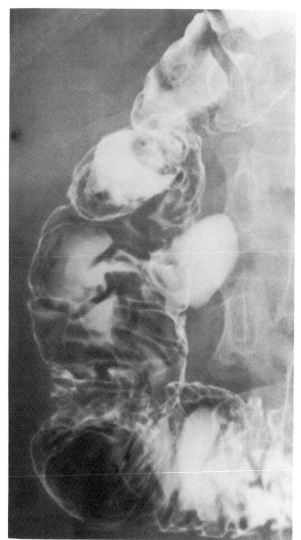

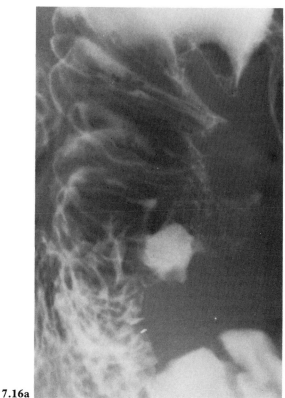

7.16a

7.16b

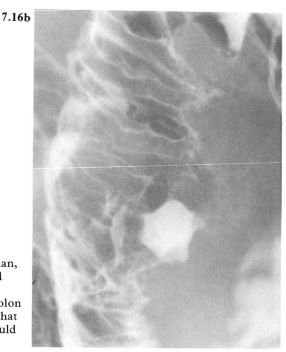

7.15 **Duodenal diverticulum** A medium-sized diverticulum is shown on a *double-contrast* view of the descending duodenum

7.16 **Carcinoma ulcerating the descending duodenum** a, b The patient, a 72-year-old woman, was admitted to hospital with haematemesis and melaena. She had been operated on five months previously when a carcinoma of the ascending colon which was invading the duodenum was found; that part of the tumour adherent to the duodenum could not be resected

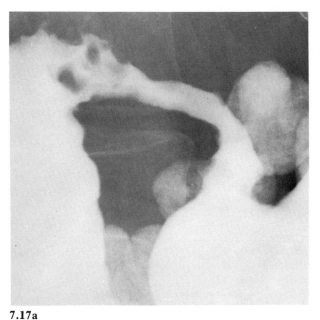

7.17a

7.17b

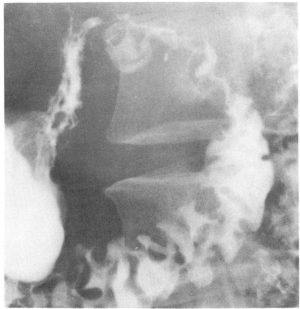

7.17c

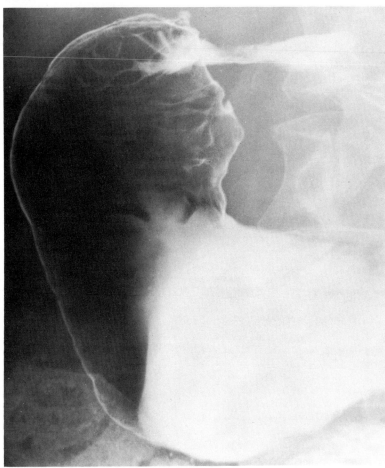

7.17 Crohn's disease of the duodenum a A narrowed segment, 10 cm in length, involving the gastric antrum, the duodenal cap and the proximal part of the descending duodenum is outlined with barium. b The remaining part of the descending duodenum is demonstrated on a *double-contrast* view and it appears normal. c Gross narrowing of the remainder of the duodenum is seen, causing obstruction.

The patient presented with vomiting and weight loss. Crohn's disease was suspected on the basis of this examination and the diagnosis was confirmed at operation

7.18a

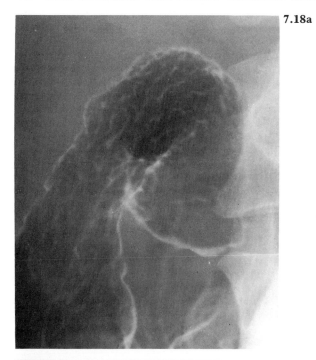

7.18b

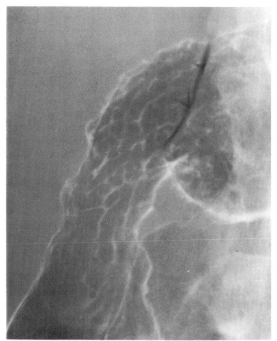

7.18c

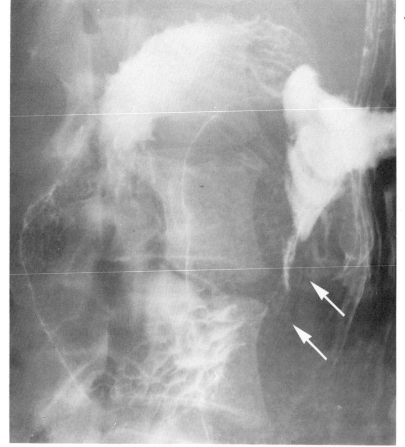

7.18 **Crohn's disease of the duodenum** a, b *Double-contrast* views show a 'cobblestone' pattern in the duodenal cap and the proximal part of the descending duodenum. c The distal part of the descending duodenum is relatively spared but there is marked involvement of the transverse duodenum with stricture formation (arrows). The patient, who was known to have Crohn's disease of the duodenum and ileum, was admitted with abdominal pain and vomiting. A gastro-jejunostomy was carried out to by-pass the stricture

7.19 **Crohn's disease with ileo-duodenal and ileo-ileal fistula formation** in a 22-year-old female known to have Crohn's disease of the ileum. a Duodeno-ileal fistula; the duodenum itself does not appear to be involved with Crohn's disease. b After a short interval a second fistula was also outlined, thought to represent an ileo-colic fistula. At operation Crohn's disease of the distal ileum and the right hemicolon was found. Fistulae from the terminal ileum to a more proximal segment of ileum and to the third part of the duodenum were identified. Histological examination of the resected specimen showed that the duodenum itself was free of Crohn's disease

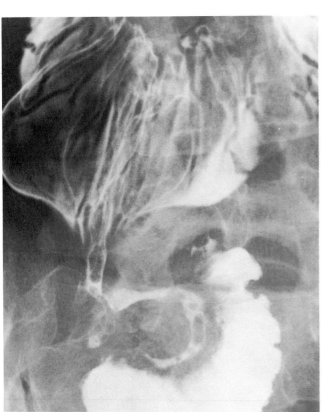

7.19a

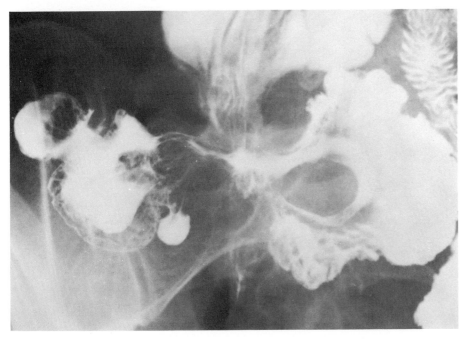

7.19b

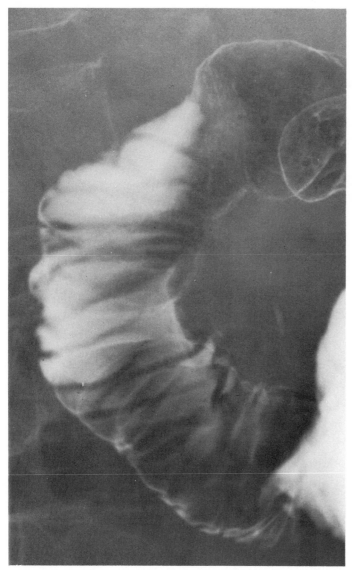

7.20 Carcinoma of the head of the pancreas A mass is shown indenting the concave aspect of the descending duodenum over a short segment at the site of the ampulla of Vater. At operation carcinoma of the head of the pancreas was found

8 Upper Gastrointestinal Bleeding

A number of workers have in recent years claimed that fibre-optic endoscopy is superior to barium radiology in upper gastrointestinal haemorrhage (Allen *et al.* 1973; Cotton *et al.* 1973; Hoare 1975). Their reports were based, however, on retrospective studies which compared the findings at endoscopy with those on opaque-type barium meal examinations. More recently the results of a prospective randomized study have been published in which endoscopy and double-contrast radiology, involving 318 patients admitted with upper gastrointestinal bleeding, have been compared (Dronfield *et al.* 1977). The diagnostic yield was higher in the endoscopy group but there was no difference between the two groups in management or survival. The accuracy of the findings when judged independently at operation and/or necropsy was also similar in the two groups. The authors concluded that early endoscopy is not essential where there is an adequate radiological service.

Angiography is a useful diagnostic procedure (Irving & Northfield 1976) particularly so when there is profuse, continuous bleeding, where the presence of a large amount of blood in the stomach is likely to obscure the field at endoscopic or barium studies. The presence of barium in the stomach or the intestines makes it impossible to carry out adequate angiography. Barium studies should not be carried out when there is evidence of active bleeding before the question of performing angiography has been considered.

Evidence of active bleeding may appear on the radiographs obtained at a double-contrast barium meal examination as a circle of non-opaque blood around the ulcer crater displacing barium — the 'halo sign' — or by blood mixed with barium flowing away from the bleeding point — the 'laval flow' pattern (Scott-Harden 1975). The bleeding point in the ulcer may be identified as a translucent defect in the barium-filled crater caused by a jet of blood coming from the bleeding vessel in the base. In some cases dilution of barium in the actual ulcer crater may be the feature that identifies the site of bleeding. The site of recent bleeding may also be identified by a small well-defined radiolucent defect in the barium-filled ulcer crater due to the presence of a plug of thrombus on the artery from which the bleeding has occurred (Potvliege *et al.* 1963). This appearance was first reported in 1932 by Berg and is often referred to as 'Bergs nodule'. Six cases were described by Åkerlund (1939) as 'stopper-shaped vascular defects' in ulcer niches.

References

Åkerlund Å. (1939) *Radiology,* **33**, 203

Allen H. M., Block M. A. & Schuman B. M. (1973) *Arch. Surg.,* **106**, 450

Berg H. H. (1932) *Fortschr. Roentgenstr.,* **46**, 147

Cotton P. B., Rosenberg M. T., Waldram R. P. L. &
Axon A. T. R. (1973) *Br. med. J.*, **2**, 505

Dronfield M. W., McIllmurray M. B., Ferguson R.,
Atkinson M. & Langman M. J. S. (1977) *Lancet*, **1**,
1167

Hoare A. M. (1975) *Br. med. J.*, **1**, 27

Irving J. D. & Northfield T. C. (1976) *Br. med. J.*, **1**,
929

Potvliege R., Engelholm J. & Potvliege D. P.
(1963) *J. Belge Radiol.*, **46**, 346

Scott-Harden W. G. (1975) In *Topics in
Gastroenterology, 3* (Ed. Truelove S. C. &
Goodman M. J.) Oxford: Blackwell Scientific
Publications

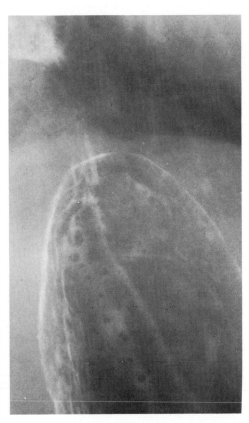

8.1 A **Mallory-Weiss tear**, about 1·5 cm in length, shown at the cardio-oesophageal junction; it was also seen at endoscopy

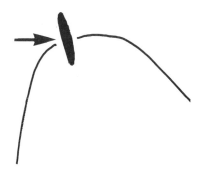

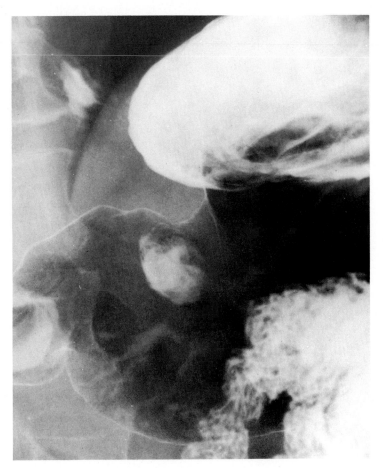

8.2 **Bleeding gastric ulcer** A *double-contrast* view of the stomach shows a large posterior-wall lesser curve ulcer containing blood and barium. Barium diluted by blood is seen flowing away from the crater, the 'laval flow' pattern, indicating that active bleeding is taking place

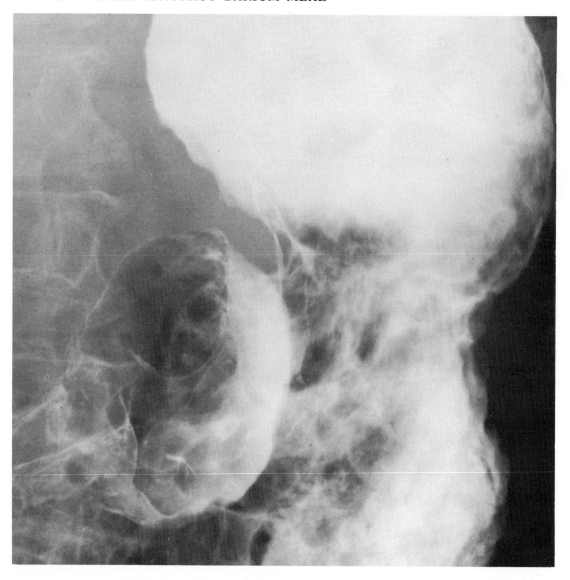

8.3 Bleeding gastric ulcer A giant lesser-curve gastric ulcer, 8 cm × 6 cm, is shown; it contains air and blood mixed with barium. The patient, an 81-year-old woman, collapsed and died 10 hours later following a further episode of bleeding. Autopsy confirmed the presence of a giant gastric ulcer

8.4a

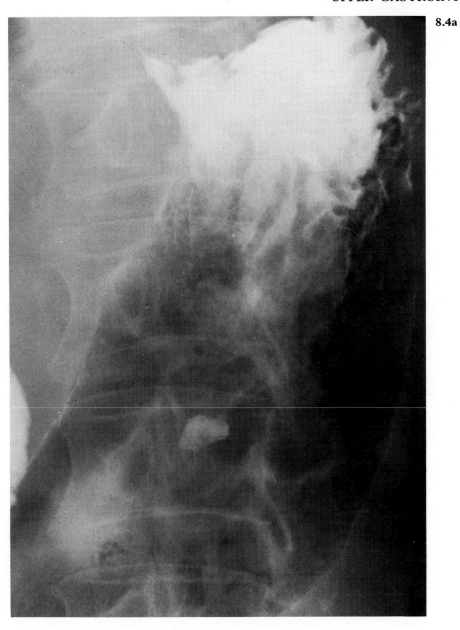

8.4 Bleeding gastric ulcer *Double-contrast* views a, b, c show a gastric ulcer with evidence of active bleeding. Blood spurting from a bleeding point in the base of the ulcer crater is seen as a small radiolucent defect. (*continued overleaf*)

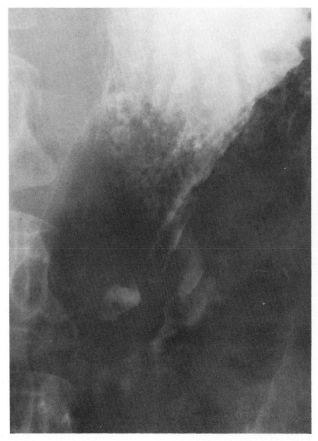

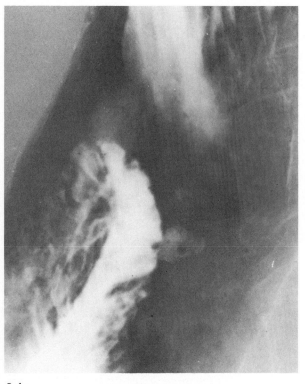

8.4c

8.4b

8.4 (*continued*) Radiolucent blood is also seen forming a circular shadow around the ulcer, the 'halo sign', and blood is diluting the barium in the stomach. The bleeding stopped and the ulcer healed following medical treatment

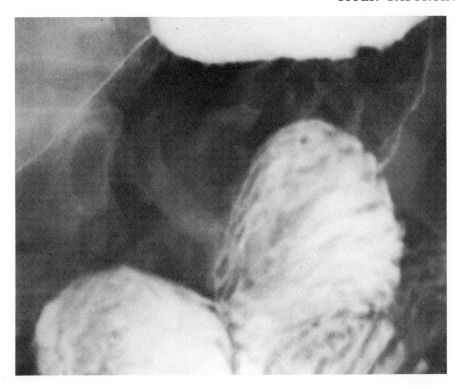

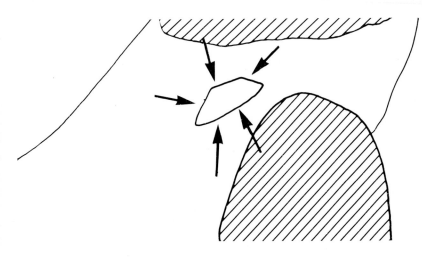

8.5 Bleeding gastric ulcer The ulcer is only faintly outlined as blood in the crater has diluted the barium. At endoscopy a large blood clot was seen adhering to the wall of the stomach at the site of the ulcer crater

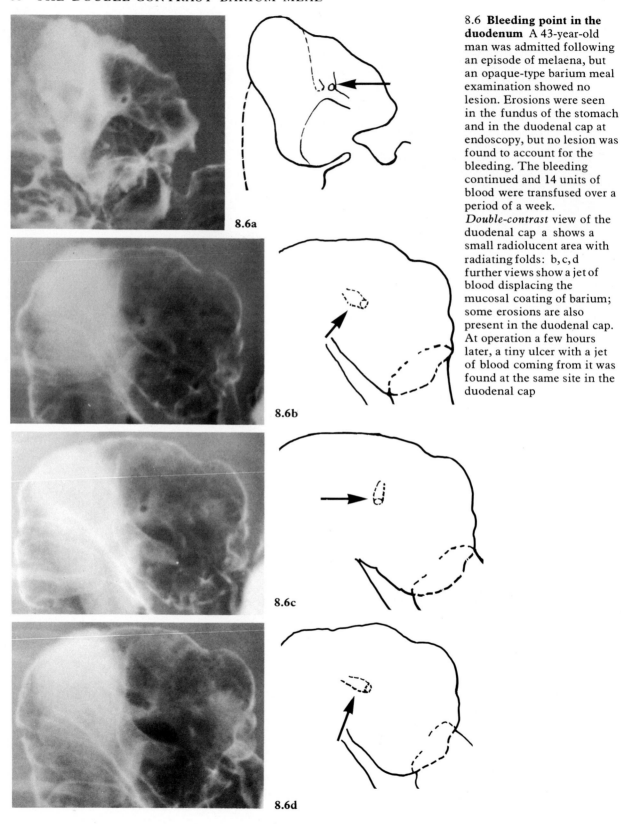

8.6a

8.6b

8.6c

8.6d

8.6 Bleeding point in the duodenum A 43-year-old man was admitted following an episode of melaena, but an opaque-type barium meal examination showed no lesion. Erosions were seen in the fundus of the stomach and in the duodenal cap at endoscopy, but no lesion was found to account for the bleeding. The bleeding continued and 14 units of blood were transfused over a period of a week.

Double-contrast view of the duodenal cap a shows a small radiolucent area with radiating folds: b, c, d further views show a jet of blood displacing the mucosal coating of barium; some erosions are also present in the duodenal cap. At operation a few hours later, a tiny ulcer with a jet of blood coming from it was found at the same site in the duodenal cap

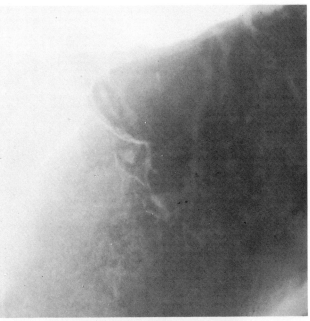

8.7 **Gastric ulcer** A shallow gastric ulcer is seen with a small blood clot in the centre. Following a further bleed the patient was operated on and the findings confirmed

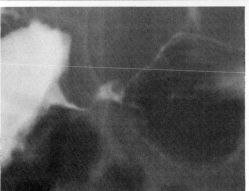

8.8 **Duodenal ulcer with 'Berg's nodule'** in a 73-year-old female patient admitted following episodes of dizziness and weakness caused by melaena; her haemoglobin was 5·6 g/100 ml. Endoscopy was carried out shortly after admission: no lesion was seen in the stomach but the pylorus was constricted and the endoscope would not pass into the duodenum. The *double-contrast* radiograph shows a duodenal ulcer with a translucent defect in the crater due to thrombus at the bleeding site — 'Berg's nodule'. There is also narrowing of the pylorus and of the base of the duodenal cap.
Laparotomy was carried out and a postérior duodenal ulcer was oversewn; a pyloroplasty and a truncal vagotomy were also carried out

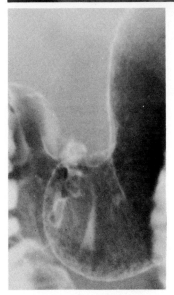

8.9 **Antral ulcer with 'Berg's nodule'** A gastric ulcer, with surrounding oedema, is shown on the lesser curve aspect of the gastric antrum. A radiolucent defect in the ulcer, due to thrombus, indicates that this was the site of bleeding. A shallow mucosal ulcer and erosions are also present

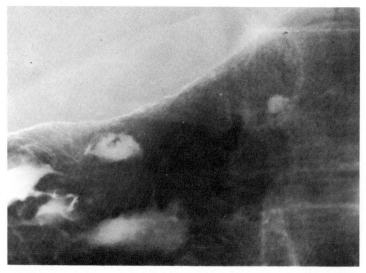

8.10a

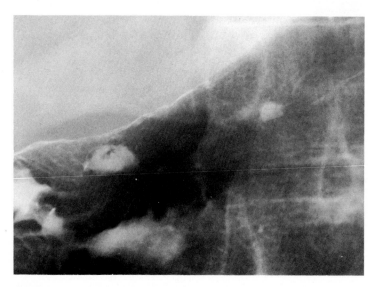

8.10b

8.10 **Gastric ulcers and 'Berg's nodule'** a, b Two gastric ulcers are
shown in a patient who was admitted with melaena. An irregular
translucent filling defect in the larger crater is due to the presence of a
blood clot — 'Berg's nodule'. The patient responded to conservative
treatment

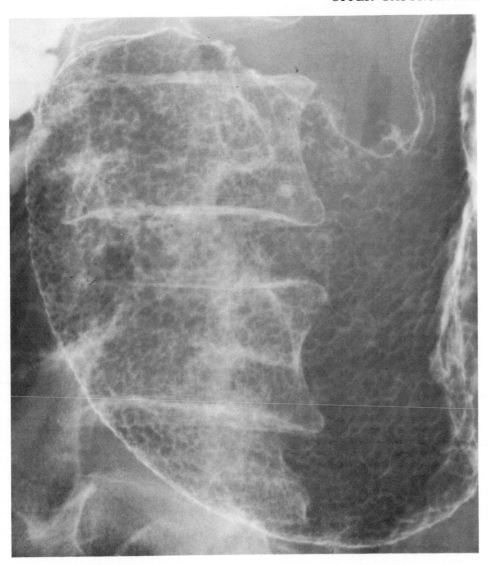

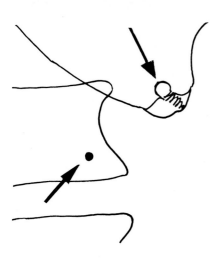

8.11 **Gastric ulcers and 'Berg's nodule'** Two small gastric ulcers are shown, one at the incisura angularis containing a radiolucent defect, 'Berg's nodule', and the other near the lesser curve aspect of the antrum. Endoscopy was carried out 24 hours later but the blood clot could not be seen because of oedema around the neck of the crater

Index